Health.   SCB

PENGUIN BOOKS
MIXED MESSAGES

Brigid McConville is an author and journalist specializing in health
and women's issues. Born in 1956, she was educated at Trinity
College, Dublin, and the University of California, Berkeley. She
began writing freelance for the Irish national press before moving
to London to work for *Business Traveller* magazine. She was runner-
up in the 1982 Catherine Pakenham Award with a study of
prostitution in Bangkok, and then went on to work for *Woman*
magazine. Her nine non-fiction books include *Women Under the
Influence: Alcohol and its Impact*, *Sisters* and *Mad To Be a Mother*. She
contributes features to many national newspapers and magazines,
including *The Times*, the *Independent*, the *Daily Telegraph*, *She* and
Marie Claire. Brigid McConville lives in Somerset with her partner
and their two young children.

with best wishes to Gill

Brigid McConville

Mixed Messages

OUR BREASTS IN OUR LIVES

Brigid McConville

PENGUIN BOOKS

PENGUIN BOOKS

Published by the Penguin Group
Penguin Books Ltd, 27 Wrights Lane, London W8 5TZ, England
Penguin Books USA Inc., 375 Hudson Street, New York, New York 10014, USA
Penguin Books Australia Ltd, Ringwood, Victoria, Australia
Penguin Books Canada Ltd, 10 Alcorn Avenue, Toronto, Ontario, Canada M4V 3B2
Penguin Books (NZ) Ltd, 182–190 Wairau Road, Auckland 10, New Zealand

Penguin Books Ltd, Registered Offices: Harmondsworth, Middlesex, England

First published 1994
10 9 8 7 6 5 4 3 2 1

The publisher wishes to thank Jonathan Cape for permission
to reproduce extracts from Philip Roth's book, *The Breast*

Typeset by Datix International Limited, Bungay, Suffolk
Printed in England by Clays Ltd, St Ives plc
Typeset in 10/13.5 pt Monophoto Photina

To John, Maeve and Arthur, my bosom companions

Contents

the breast • Looking after your breasts • How to check
your breasts

List of figures

Acknowledgements

Hundreds of people, in many different ways, have contributed to this book and I would like to thank them all.

I am particularly grateful to Professor Barry Gusterson and his colleagues Ros Eeles, Judy Deacon and Julian Peto at the Institute of Cancer Research. They answered my questions with care and read my manuscript for accuracy. Professor Robert Mansel and Charlene Bargeron of the Breast Care Campaign also provided me with invaluable information on breast health and double-checked my facts.

Gabrielle Palmer, Sheila Kitzinger, Chloe Fisher, Mary Renfrew and Sally Inch helped me enormously with their ideas and expertise – and also checked the manuscript for accuracy. Dora Henschel, Pat Last and Andrea Whalley gave generously of their time and knowledge as did many individuals from Breast Cancer Care. I am also grateful to the Bristol Cancer Help Centre, Dr Paul Brown and Alan Riley who gave me very useful advice and information.

Special thanks to the following who, between them, contributed ideas, contacts, sources and – above all – their own experiences: Lizzie Cox, Gwen Webber, Avril Silk, Madeleine Morey, Libby Lisgo, Ruth Lester, Peggy Walker, Sue Watling, Charlotte Webster, Maureen Beck, Judy Skinner, Alison Alcock, Donna Pollak, Jill Jones, Gilly Lee, Sarah Howard, Sue Duffen, Caroline

Buck, Sue Jenkins, Sarah Jervis, Hilary Grayson, Dionne Villani and Alison Hahloe. Thanks also to Tessa Shaw and Christina Ward Pearce for their film *The Tip of the Iceberg*, and to Anne Dibble and Gilly Model for describing the role of the breast care nurse.

My sisters Fran, Lucy and Emily McConville gave me their support and help, while my parents Mike and Beryl McConville and my partner John Shearlaw kept me supplied with essential cuttings and books. Special thanks also to Dr Richard Lee, for his invaluable practical help and cheerful interest.

My thanks to those many women I interviewed who remain anonymous, as well as to the women of Taunton and District NCT, East Dulwich NCT, the Association of Breastfeeding Mothers in Taunton, *Justwomen* magazine and the women students at Wellington Community College in Somerset. Heartfelt thanks also to Clare Bainbridge who rescued me from computer darkness, to Madonna Duffy for her patience and to Margaret Bluman, a discerning and supportive editor.

Introduction

I first came across the subject of breasts when I reported for the *Independent* on a new telephone helpline set up by the Breast Care Campaign in 1992. Women, I had been told, were ringing up the helpline to pour out their secret woes, and to express deep anxieties, often for the first time.

Many had been to their GP about a breast lump, but had come away still worried and none the wiser, having met with dismissive or patronizing attitudes. Some doctors seemed to know as little about breasts as they knew about women's feelings for their breasts.

Who, then, *did* understand about breasts? I looked for psycho-sexual research studies and British 'experts' who could make sense of the reasons behind all this confusion. But in Britain – in contrast to other countries – we don't seem able to take breasts seriously. Other countries have international conferences on breast health where they discuss the breast in the spheres of art, relationships and medicine. This country has Benny Hill, page three and burly pantomime dames with balloons up their jumpers.

I turned to the real 'experts' on breasts: women. In interviews with over a hundred women – in groups, individually and through organizations like the Breast Care Campaign, the National Childbirth Trust and the Association of Breastfeeding Mothers – I was told about the significance of breasts in their lives.

They remembered acute teenage self-consciousness; men's remarks; anxieties about 'measuring up' as women. They talked of their fears and experiences of breast cancer; of the highs and lows of breastfeeding; of sex, pornography, cosmetic surgery and, all too often, of bad experiences with doctors.

I spoke to some young women in their teens. They tended to be on the defensive against boys at school who defined them in terms of breast size, calling them 'jugs' or 'wall'. I spoke to some older women with memories of being pushed into conical bras and regrets about becoming 'droopy'. But mostly I spoke to women in their thirties or forties who had reached a confident acceptance of their own breasts – but only after years of ambivalence.

For many women breasts are a battleground, laid claim to by men, medics and – occasionally – babies. Advertisers, porn and pin-up merchants, fashion designers, plastic surgeons and artificial milk manufacturers all struggle for control over this female place where the maternal and the erotic coincide.

But the chief contenders are men. I wanted to ask men – how do you really feel about breasts? What is this obsession all about? Men in other cultures are not so fixated by this body part. In other times, other places, men have focussed their erotic interest on stomachs, thighs, bottoms, even the nape of the neck.

But in asking men direct questions about breasts you generally get a lot of excitement and hooting and that's the end of it. Men tend not to analyse and discuss their feelings in the same way that many women do. The local Rotarians thought they might talk to me, but wanted to know what I looked like first. I doubted our discussions would be fruitful.

I tried a questionnaire for men, but the answers weren't very revealing. I did quiz some individual men, but the conversation turned quickly into a kind of shopping list of favoured breast shapes and sizes.

But just because most men haven't worked out what they feel about breasts doesn't mean that it isn't apparent. The indications are all around us – on television, in the tabloids, in daily chit-chat, in novels and films. Behind the banter and the slang is tremendous need and desire (for sex, for comfort) mixed with fear (of women, of the power of the maternal). It is a volatile combination with sometimes nasty results.

One of these is male hostility to breastfeeding. More than one midwife told me that men's jealousy was the main reason why women in this country give up breastfeeding early. There is a powerful feeling that breasts are for sex and that, therefore, they 'belong' to a woman's husband or partner.

Another nasty result is widespread ignorance of breasts. I had never seen a diagram of the breast before researching this book, and few of the women I interviewed had either. None of my interviewees remembered learning about breasts at school. Few women regularly examined their breasts either.

Few of us ever see another woman's breasts, except for the phoney 'perfect' breasts of young models to which we feel unfavourably compared. We think we live in liberated times, but there is a curfew on breastfeeding women and a mother who bares her breast in public still risks humiliating banishment – often to a toilet.

And for women whose breasts develop medical problems, treatments have a distinctly punitive feel. Women are semi-stripped, their breasts are squashed between hard plates for X-ray and punctured by needles, without anaesthetic.

Years of campaigning by American women drew attention to the fact that many surgeons were still doing mastectomies for breast cancer long after it was shown that less drastic operations were equally effective.

In Britain, too, the quality of care for women with breast

diseases has met with fierce criticism, from women and doctors alike. Britain has fewer specialist breast cancer surgeons than any other Western country.

Successive governments have done little to fight what is the biggest killer of women in their middle years, and we have the highest death rate in the world from breast cancer. Under the circumstances, the spirit and the courage of the women who describe their experiences of breast cancer in this book are very impressive.

One reason why so many British women die is that we come forward for medical treatment at a dangerously late stage. Why? We come back full circle to our culture's breast taboos. Breasts mean 'sex', therefore many of us are uncomfortable about exposing our breasts to the scrutiny and prodding of our (mostly male) doctors. Breasts – in the cancer context – also mean 'death', and this is a society which can hardly bear to mention the word 'cancer'. No wonder the helplines are busy.

There are some good books on breastfeeding and on breast health. There are excellent support groups for women with breast cancer and for women who want to breastfeed. But this is the first book to bring these subjects together and to link them to the cultural attitudes which so profoundly affect us all. I hope that when we have understood the reasons for the battles, we can begin to make peace.

Brigid McConville, 1993

1
Living with breasts:
women's experience

By any other name?

Talking of breasts, we have an immediate problem: the language. Breast is a good, honest word – and yet many of us are intensely uncomfortable about using it. But then this part of the body has many powerful meanings which can be disturbingly incompatible. 'Breast' can mean eroticism, as the focus of excitement between lovers. It can mean motherhood, as in the swollen breasts of pregnancy and the milk-giving breasts of the woman who suckles her baby. And it has medical meanings too, as the site of pain, of fatal and 'unmentionable' illness. It is a word that spans our great taboos – sex and death – taking in motherhood along the way.

And how should we use the word? If it is the right word to use to a doctor, might the whiff of the surgery not linger when we use it with a lover? If we use it with a lover, does the erotic meaning not hang in the air when we talk about feeding babies with our breasts? The porn and pin-up connotations also lurk in the back of our minds to muddy the other meanings with smuttiness, embarrassment and even guilt.

As a result many women won't use the word 'breast' at all. Particularly for people of the older generation, or for people brought up to think of sex as somehow 'dirty', breast is akin to a dirty word:

My mother wouldn't call a breast a breast. She called it her 'chest'.

My mother does say 'breasts' but she practically spits it out: 'Brreasstss!'.

Yet what are the alternatives? 'Bosom' is quite affectionate and dignified but it also seems very old-fashioned, Victorian, and certainly sexless. 'Bust' is also sexually neutral and rather dated, suggesting the kind of large, monolithic shelf that elderly aunties used to carry around under their twin sets. Indeed, some women describe their 'bust' (singular) as 'the shelf', which is not only singular, but is 'out there' and detached from the owner.

Then there is the slang – tits, boobs, knockers. Women are equally uncomfortable with these, and many of us resent them intensely:

I can't bear to hear men talk of 'tits' and 'knockers', when what they are talking about is something lovely, rounded and sensual.

Tit and boob are belittling words. Boob also means 'stupid' or 'mistake', while to 'make a tit of yourself' means doing something really foolish.

In his *Dictionary of Slang and Unconventional English*, Eric Partridge records that 'tit' once meant 'the female pudend' ('pudend', from the Latin word for 'shame', is how dictionaries denote women's genitalia). Then 'tit' came to mean 'girl' or 'harlot', before its modern sense of 'breast' or 'nipple'.

There are also ugly connotations to the word nipple in various languages. According to Sheila Kitzinger, who travels widely to lecture on breastfeeding, several European languages call the nipple a 'breast wart'. 'Wart' has implications of witchcraft as well as ugliness.

There is another kind of slang for breasts – the comical,

nursery-rhyme type. Words like 'jallopies', 'baloobas', 'montezu-mas'. They sound wobbly, bouncy, round and funny. You can hear the onomatopoeic wiggle – and the giggle. One of the first jokes children hear at school is about a woman looking for her dog, who is called 'Titswobble'. (Q: Have you seen my Titswobble? A: No, but I'd like to!)

There are other schoolboyish, bragging words like 'knockers', 'melons' and 'stonkers', inevitably prefixed by 'huge' or 'gigantic'. In a class of fourteen- and fifteen-year-old boys and girls who were asked to come up with words for 'breasts' (part of a sex education course in a Bridgwater school), this was the result: *lemons, balloons, footballs, jellies, melons, whoppers, knockers, bazook-ers, tits, toys, fried eggs, bee stings, sand dunes, boobs, jugs, tools, bits, pancakes, milk floats, lumps, dust caps* and *John Wayne's saddlebags*.

But most women don't want mocking, bragging, joking or insulting words to describe this cherished, intimate part of them-selves. These words have no dignity and no beauty. The word breast is still the most direct word that we have. Yet it doesn't sound like *our* word. It is too formal and functional. And it is also too sexy, even smutty.

Over and again, while working on this book, I found myself in difficulty with language. People simply weren't comfortable with the *name* of my subject matter. This became a familiar dialogue:

> 'I hear you are writing a book. What is it about?'
> (Me) 'Breasts.'
> (Pause) 'Breasts? Ah!' (Pause. Glance at the ground. In older people a clearing of the throat. In younger people a kind of strangled giggle.)

Each time I had to resist the impulse to justify myself, as if this subject were somehow suspect or silly or salacious. Yet it would be only a matter of minutes before women were telling me vivid stories of their experiences – of being big-breasted or small-breasted, of men's remarks, of their fear at finding breast lumps. Men were fascinated too, although rather pink-cheeked about it all.

So at times I have longed for a different word, a neutral, a 'safe' word. But the breast isn't a 'safe' subject; it is a highly charged and taboo subject. Perhaps when we have aired some of the tensions surrounding breasts, when we have talked about them a bit more and challenged some of the taboos, we will be able to use the word 'breast' again without embarrassment.

Whose breasts are they anyway?

We live with them day to day. We are, literally, physically and emotionally attached to them. So why do so many women express the feeling that our breasts are a battleground?

It is a theme which crops up again and again when women talk about breasts. In the street, at work, in the doctor's surgery, in breastfeeding children, women are made to feel that their breasts are somehow separate from themselves – and that their rightful owners are in fact men:

> Men call themselves 'tit men' or 'leg men' – as if women were divided into separate bits.

> Men judge and feel they have a right to judge our breasts. They make quite gratuitous comments, everywhere you go.

> I don't think most women think about their breasts except through

the eyes of men. We are taught to picture ourselves like that – as
men see us.

On one level we know that they are, of course, *our* breasts. We
have our own feelings about them, ranging from pride and
pleasure to dislike and shame. They are a part of our identity,
affecting our health, self-esteem and sexuality.

Yet, on another level, our breasts have been subject to a
massive male takeover bid. They are no longer unique, integral
aspects of ourselves. We see breasts daily as free-floating parts
that can be pictured and parodied in all sorts of ways, from porn
to breast kitsch.

Novelty shops sell blow-up bath pillows and plastic strap-on
falsies shaped as breasts. There are drinking cups with nipples to
sip from. Hot water bottles with breasts, 'joke' dolls with pop-out
breasts, hats, T-shirts – you name it, it comes in 'boob' form.

Fashion has added to this sense of breasts as things apart
from us. The bras and stars of fifties Hollywood lifted and
separated breasts from each other, but also from women. They
were breasts that came into a room ahead of a woman, almost
under their own steam. And again in the eighties and nineties
fashion has been setting breasts apart, thrusting them forwards
with corsets and Wonderbras, parodying them in Gaultier's
stuck-on cones, emphasizing them with Vivienne Westwood's
externally-worn bras (she has said it was a man's – Malcolm
Maclaren's – idea).

And of course there are the ever-present images. The breast-
implanted supermodels, the page-three girls, the soft porn mags,
the *Sunday Sport*'s mega breasts, the Hollywood cleavages, the
calendar girls and adverts – even the cardboard nudes under
the pub's peanuts. Sometimes it seems as if breasts are keeping
the wheels of commerce turning all by themselves.

Yet these female 'parts' are not like ordinary women's breasts. They are models' breasts, uniformly young, pert, uptilted and pre-fertile. Most of us don't have breasts like that, and so they make us feel that our bodies are never as good as other women's bodies.

Magazines, newspapers and films very rarely show the reality of breasts – unless they are featuring poverty-stricken women from the developing world. Even when it comes to serious and responsible articles about breast cancer, the pictures are of young women's breasts, despite the fact that young women are not at risk.

Gérard Depardieu, the actor, has complained that when he tells women 'you have beautiful breasts', they don't welcome his comments. Wouldn't it be nice to be able to accept that sort of remark as it may well have been intended, simply as a compliment, as pleasing as 'you have a beautiful face'?

Unfortunately for us, and for Gérard, as long as we are made to feel that our breasts are a male fiefdom women will react to such comments like resentful colonials. Women – and men – are forced into the difficult position where *whatever* men say about breasts will feel like a put-down.

This has profound consequences for women's health care, because when doctors talk about breasts (and doctors are mostly men), women are hearing yet more male assessment. Whether he is aware of it or not, the doctor who says 'no need to worry about your breasts' risks sounding patronizing or dismissive. The doctor who says, 'you will have no trouble breastfeeding', risks his patient thinking that this is a comment on her figure.

Some men have made it worse for all of us by behaving as if they have the right to touch us as well as to stare and comment on our breasts. Many women have stories to tell of men walking along the pavement or standing near them on public transport –

or even at work – who have grabbed or pinched their breast. Many of us have experienced the unsolicited, unwelcome breast grope or nipple tweak:

> I was walking home from the shops and I noticed this young lad coming towards me. As he went past he just reached out a hand and grabbed my breast. Then he just kept on walking.

Most commonly these are annoying incidents that make us feel upset, vulnerable or just plain angry for a time. But they can also be part of a more extreme abuse: the driving instructor who gropes his learner drivers; the doctor who touches up his vulnerable patients. Women who eventually report such incidents say they were initially too shocked to do anything about them.

Perhaps if we felt more connected to our breasts, more like their proud and rightful owners, we would object more immediately when men laid hands upon them. But even the way our breasts have developed – out and away from us, and often very quickly – contributes to this sense of not being in control.

Most of us get used to this feeling of separateness. We learn to live with our breasts, sometimes stoically, sometimes affectionately. As one woman put it:

> It's as if our breasts have their own identities, as if they are separate characters – rather like men's 'willies'.

Handing them over to doctors

When it comes to health care, too, women say they feel as if their breasts don't belong to them. The days when women would go under an anaesthetic expecting to have a biopsy, only to wake without a breast, have gone. But the medical tendency to treat the breasts as interesting organs, rather than an intrinsic part of a woman, has not yet disappeared. Women complain that doctors talk about their breasts as if they weren't present, as if their breasts were a disembodied phenomenon (see Chapter Eight).

The literature which gives women's views on breast surgery is full of stories like this one, from a woman being told by doctors that she needed a mastectomy (from *Disorderly Breasts*, by Sarah Boston and Jill Louw):

> Finally he found this note and then got a pen out of his pocket and said, 'That's the breast that is coming off', and put a cross on the breast.

And in this story from the *Daily Telegraph* (4.12.92):

> A woman who was shopping around for a breast reduction operation walked out of a consulting room after the doctor pulled up her bra and – without a by-your-leave – began sketching in new nipple sites with a felt pen.

Women complain about being expected to 'hand over' their breasts once they consult a doctor (see Chapter Eight). They talk about the 'breast cancer conveyor belt', as if they have no control over what happens to their breasts. Above all, they say they aren't given enough information or choices about treatments for breast disorders.

It doesn't have to be like that. One of the purposes of this book is to give women information so that we can make the best choices – and to give us back a sense of control over our breasts.

Move over, baby

But perhaps more than in any other arena, it is in breastfeeding that women experience their breasts as a battleground. It can be difficult enough for women when their 'sex symbols' (as this society sees them) are turned so rapidly into baby-feeding organs. In a sense, through pregnancy and childbirth a woman's body has already been taken over by another person. But the stress piles on when men get jealous of 'their' woman's breasts, 'their breasts', being used by the new infant:

> The other morning I turned on the television to discover the studio audience on a chat-show busily discussing breasts. I had my nipper on the nipple at the time, so I was simultaneously distracted and attentive when I heard a horrid, weaselly-looking fellow saying that he didn't like his wife to breastfeed. Why? 'I find it quite repulsive', he said, 'and, quite honestly, I think her breasts belong to me.' (*She* magazine, July 1992)

It's unusual to hear a man declare his sense of ownership so blatantly, but a midwife of many years' experience has told me that this is *the* major reason why women give up breastfeeding – or don't even start.

From the 'weaselly fellow's' point of view, it's obvious. He doesn't want to see another's hands touching what he wants to touch, another's mouth sucking on what he wants to suck.

But why should we accept such claims to our bodies? Men may be interested in our breasts. They may be passionate, fixated or utterly obsessed. But they remain our bodies, our breasts. It is up to us to decide if we want to breastfeed. It is up to us to choose when we breastfeed, how often and for how long. We can, if we are aware of the pressures, reclaim control of this disputed region of our bodies. The purpose of this book is to raise that awareness and help women make those choices for themselves.

Waiting for them to grow

Are there any of us who can't remember the time when our breasts arrived – or at least, the time when they were *supposed to* arrive? It is a time of such exquisite self-consciousness that chance remarks from friends, parents or siblings are never forgotten, and passing events that focussed attention on our bodies are etched in the memory:

> When I was ten I slipped in the bath and I remember feeling just the faintest quiver of flesh. Bemused, I re-enacted the same slip. It was the strangest ripple. Barely noticeable. Then the realization slowly dawned. My breasts had arrived. (Nilgin Yusuf, *Cosmopolitan*)

> I can still remember forcing Mum to buy me a teen bra size 28AA when I was fourteen, only to discover that it was at least two sizes too big. The humiliation! I was convinced that some day I would wake up and find my boobs had miraculously grown overnight. They never did. (Antonella Lazzeri in the *Sun*, 9.10.92)

Girls at this age are acutely conscious of who is 'developing' and who is not:

> I remember going on holiday with two schoolfriends who I thought were 'developed' while I was 'flat'. I sat all summer on the beach,

hunched over to hide my chest. Recently I found a holiday snap of the three of us, and what did I see? Two fat girls and one slim one, hunched over. But that's not how I saw us at the time.

And because they know just how tender feelings can be when it comes to breasts, some girls will use remarks about breasts when they want to be nasty:

> The girls at school used to say to me – 'Look down. Can you see your toes? Of course you can. There's nothing in the way.' I used to watch all the younger ones filing into assembly every day. I wasn't watching their faces – I was looking at their breasts to see if any of them had grown bigger than me. It was awful. I have got over that feeling. I now like having small breasts. But it has taken about twenty years!

> I went to a new school when I was fourteen and immediately ran into trouble with the pecking order. The girls soon found a way of putting me in my place. There was a girl in our class whose status – although low in academic terms – was gigantic when it came to her looks. The other girls told me that her breasts were perfect: rounded, firm as half-melons and placed high up on her chest. They measured her from shoulder to nipple. Then they measured me from shoulder to nipple. My measurement was inches longer. The other girls were triumphant: I had been measured against the ideal, and found wanting! So there.

Boys, too, can use remarks about breasts to put girls down. A fifteen-year-old friend tells me that the boys in her school openly call girls with big breasts 'jugs'. Girls with small breasts are called 'wall' or 'bee-sting'.

Rite of passage

This time of developing breasts can also be a crucial point in relationships between parents and daughters. Here are the first physical signs of a little girl turning into a woman, of an emerging sexuality. All the old taboos are being stirred. How will the father feel about his newly sexual daughter? How will the mother feel about having another pair of breasts – younger, firmer, closer to the stereotyped 'ideal' – protruding into her territory?

> My daughter's breasts developed astonishingly quickly. It was as if they grew about an inch a day. And they kept growing and growing. I began to worry that they might not stop. Of course they did stop, but they are now quite a bit bigger than mine. I didn't really know what to feel. I made some comments to my husband, but he refused to be drawn on the subject.

> I used to wear a Fairisle jumper a lot when I was about fourteen, and I can remember my father smiling at me kindly and saying, 'Every time I see you that pattern is higher up your chest.' It was quite sweet really: he helped me feel rather pleased and proud of myself.

But sometimes there can be awkwardness, embarrassment and downright hostility at home. And when a mother takes her daughter out to buy her first bra, unworthy emotions may come out:

> I remember that horrendous first fitting. My mother put me into a size too small. It was an awful pointy thing. I went home and cut the tops off it. I'm sure that it was my mother's jealousy at work.

The American journalist Nora Ephron, writing in *Esquire* magazine twenty years ago, remembers what it was like when her friends began to 'develop' but she did not. She sat in the bath, waiting for them to grow, but they didn't:

> 'I want to buy a bra', I said to my mother one night. 'What for?' she said. My mother was really hateful about bras, and by the time my third sister had gotten to the point where she was ready to want one, my mother had worked the whole business into a comedy routine. 'Why not use a Band-Aid instead?' she would say.

> It was a source of great pride to my mother that she had never even had to wear a brassiere until she had her fourth child, and then only because her gynaecologist made her. It was incomprehensible to me that anyone could be proud of something like that. It was the 1950s for God's sake. Jane Russell. Cashmere sweaters. Couldn't my mother see that?

> 'I am too old to wear an undershirt.' Screaming. Weeping. Shouting. 'Then don't wear an undershirt', said my mother. 'But I want to buy a bra.' 'What for?'

Eventually most girls' breasts do grow. Some hate turning so obviously into a girl, losing their 'one of the boys' status (children learn very early that male is higher status than female). Others are delighted and proud of their new shape.

Some women go on hoping long into adulthood that their breasts will grow larger. Some women suffer acute unhappiness about the smallness of their breasts and eventually resort to surgery. But many small-breasted women say that, as they mature and form relationships, they come to like their breasts just as they are.

But for girls whose breasts grow to be larger than usual – whether they like their size or not – the obviousness of their measurements can become bound up with their public persona for a long time to come.

Big breasts: boon or burden?

Many of us – women and men alike – have a great affection for big breasts. From Ma Larkin to Beryl Cook, popular culture is rich with images of the ample, warm and generous 'bosom'. If we are lucky, we remember the childhood hugs and cuddles:

> All of my aunties were large-breasted women. There always seemed to be these masses of heaving bosom when I was younger. It was terribly comforting. You could lean against them, and it was warm and solid. The bras they wore were armour-like, more protective than today's bras. They seemed very secure and solid.

> I remember hugging my mum, and that feeling of laying my head against a big, gentle, warm bosom. It was lovely.

And many women enjoy having big breasts:

> I think my breasts are the best part of me. They make me feel that I am really womanly, sexy and attractive. And it pleases me that they please my husband so much.

> To be honest, I do think that my breasts are my greatest physical asset. They are quite large and I do notice that men notice them. I'm rather pleased with them all in all.

Women's breasts are growing larger on average too. In the last decade the average bust size of women in the UK has increased from 34B to 36C (*Independent on Sunday*, 12.1.92). This is because of various factors, including improved nutrition, more exercise and the effects of the Pill.

And at the beginning of the nineties, big breasts were very much in vogue (see Chapter Three). The Gossard Wonderbra with its uplift and emphasis on cleavage staged a spectacular comeback, and many catwalk models have had breast implants to make themselves look bigger.

But we are nothing if not ambivalent about breasts, and for every reason to be happy with big breasts, there are others to wish them away.

Big breasts have long been a male joke. Comedians say that 'tits are the best gag in the world'. In seaside postcards, in tabloid newspapers, on the Benny Hill and Ronnie Barker shows, big breasts are to be ogled at, pointed at, giggled at. Even when the 'jokes' are at men's expense, the recognized cue for comedy is the image of the swelling bosom.

In day-to-day life men stare at big breasts, whistle at women with big breasts – and sometimes make a grab at them. Some women do enjoy the attention, but it can be maddening to be perceived as no more than a 'big pair of knockers'. Many women suffer the hurt of being known as 'big tits' or 'the biggest boobs in town'. It can make for a lot of bad feeling towards men:

> Men don't look me in the eye when they talk to me. They seem to be mesmerized by my breasts, like rabbits in headlamps. Sometimes I feel like prodding them and saying – Oi! Snap out of it! There's a person behind this prow.

> Young men were forever fixated on my breasts. I hated it. Until I realized the power that I had – and then I used them.

> A full bosom is actually a millstone around a woman's neck: it endears her to the men who want to make their mammet of her, but she is never allowed to think that their popping eyes actually see her ... [breasts] are not part of a person, but lures slung around her neck, to be kneaded and twisted like magic putty, or mumbled and mouthed like lolly ices. (Germaine Greer, *The Female Eunuch*)

Big breasts are for barmaids. All the better to tell your troubles to, my dear. Big breasts are for bimbos, for page-three girls of little brain. In an ugly 'Griffin's Eye' cartoon (*Daily Mirror*, 29.9.92), Samantha Fox, breasts as large as the rest of her body, holds up the announcement that she is one of Britain's richest women. 'It's my singing wot done it,' reads the caption. Big breasts equals ignorant, common, coarse.

There is a widespread assumption that the bigger your cup size, the smaller your hat size:

> I remember an article in the *Guardian* – it was about fifteen years ago – which said that if you have large breasts, then the chances are your brain is not up to much. It had been scientifically investigated by educationalists that the smaller your breasts the more intelligent you were. If you had large breasts you were not likely to be terribly bright; you would make a good homemaker instead. I thought – well, tough luck for me then.

Lusty busty?

It is as if men have cornered the market on brain power. In the traditional Western dichotomy, thought belongs to male and body belongs to female. The more female you are – i.e. the bigger your breasts – the more biologically driven and sexual you are. Big-breasted women are seen as 'better at it'. The corollary is that small-breasted women are 'naturally' less responsive and less interested in sex:

> When you are big breasted, people call you 'Lusty Busty'. They

think you have more of an appetite for sex and that you enjoy it more.

It may well be true that the big-breasted woman is more attractive to some men. Certainly, Hollywood films of the forties elevated large-breasted women to the highest heights of sex-symbol stardom, making a strong impact on a whole generation. (Andrew Stanway, the psychosexual therapist and author, goes so far as to suggest that you can guess the age of a man by his views on the 'ideal' breast size: the bigger the cup, the older the man.)

But isn't it just a fact of life that big breasts are a sexual turn-on? Of course, breasts can be sexy. They are stimulating to see and to touch and to have touched. They are the visible signals of female gender in an era when many of the other traditional female signals – skirts, hairdos, lipstick – have become strictly optional.

But other times and other places haven't elevated breasts into being so overwhelmingly, exclusively, powerfully sexy as we have. Sexy as long as they stay firm, uptilted and aged eighteen. Sexy as long as they aren't feeding babies.

Masters and Johnson, in their book *Human Sexuality*, say that our attitude to breasts as sex objects is:

> not universal by any means, and in some cultures, little or no erotic importance is attached to the breasts. For example, in Japan, women traditionally bound their breasts to make them inconspicuous. Today, however, the Westernization process has brought about changes in Japan and the breasts have become rather fully eroticized.

(With, incidentally, some rather grim consequences for Japanese women. After the Second World War, as American GIs flooded into Japan, some Japanese women tried to increase their bust measurements by having silicone injections directly into their chests – risking long-term illness and disability.)

There is no evidence to suggest that breast size has any relation to a woman's interest in sex, nor to her sexual responsiveness. In fact, it seems that bigger breasts feel less sensation than smaller ones, as nerve endings are thinner on the ground. Masters and Johnson say that many women experience little sexual sensation when their breasts are caressed anyway – whatever their size.

Related to the 'lusty busty' myth is the notion that the bigger your breasts, the more dozily maternal you are – and the more able to produce milk for babies:

> The doctor looked at me when I was pregnant and said, 'Ho ho, you'll have no difficulty feeding your children.' I felt quite put down. Maybe he meant it to be a compliment. But I didn't feel it to be such. He made me feel a bit like an animal. Like a cow. Bovine.

And physically too big breasts can be quite a burden. They can interfere with the simplest events of daily life, from breast-feeding a baby to running for a bus:

> There is a certain amount of discomfort involved. They're rather droopy and it hurts to hike them up. When I'm bending over, doing something like gardening, I pop out over the top of my bra.

> Buying a bra is a major task. It could take me hours. And then there is the inconvenience of shaping dresses to fit me.

> I wished for years that I could wake up flat-chested one day. I get entangled in my own breasts. If there was a fire, the first thing I would grab would be my bra – because it's so difficult to get a comfy one.

> They were the bane of my life, those cumbersome things. Models

were always lean, lithe lovelies. No fear of their chests wibbly-wobbling or bouncing in great jelly jumps. It was also obvious that clothes hung better on a flat chest. In terms of style, two full breasts infinitely complicated matters. Anything frilly or fussy was out of the question, giving the appearance of an over-inflated rooster. No pockets over bosoms, and definitely no buttons over nipples. (Nilgin Yusuf, *Cosmopolitan*)

And sometimes, women find their big breasts a serious problem. In *The Breast*, women told Drs Andrew and Penny Stanway that:

I've wished all my life that mine were less. I went round looking at other women and thinking – oh God nobody seems to have the same sort of breasts as me. It did affect me, especially in my teens and early twenties. It made me very conscious of my body.

If only people realized how awful it is having big breasts. Men are foul to you. You get wolf-whistles from all the wrong ones. I had endless backache and neck pain and I couldn't get a bra anywhere. I really felt a freak. In the end I had to have plastic surgery. Life just wasn't worth living any more.

The guilty breast

There is another problem with having breasts – big or small – that can make women wish they didn't have them. It stems from another old sex-myth with its origins way back in the traditions of misogyny. It belongs to the realm of dark and dirty secrets about women's bodies, reflecting the age-old male fear of the 'polluting' aspects of women's sexual organs. It says that breasts are bad and will bring punishment.

Andrew and Penny Stanway almost incidentally reveal a Pandora's box of these repressive breast myths in *The Breast*, written only a decade ago:

> Breasts should never be made to seem 'dirty' or 'wrong' to a young girl – or indeed to anybody ... If a girl is made to feel sinful or wrong for allowing a boy to touch her breasts, she'll carry that guilt with her for years and possibly even for ever.

The Stanways go on to refer to the idea – as old as religion – that 'sin' manifests itself in physical sickness:

> Children should never be led to believe that breast play could lead to cancer. There is absolutely no truth in this. There is no evidence at all that any form of sexual activity (including practices in which the breasts come into contact with the penis or semen) causes cancer or any other diseases. Similarly, there's no evidence at all that powder, perfume or anything else used on the breasts does them any harm. Nipple and breast play have no effect on the progress of the menopause and can, of course, be continued after it.

The American writer Susan Love in her *Breast Book* indicates how widespread this kind of myth is:

> Many women enjoy having their breasts stroked or sucked by their lovers, but have been told that this too can lead to cancer. It can't. Breasts, after all, are made to be suckled.

One reason why these ideas are so common is that people have a deep need to find 'causes' for illness. We all want to know why we are ill – or why other people are ill – to give us some sense of understanding and control over what we fear. And when that illness is breast illness, guilt about sex is never far behind.

The psychologist Lesley Fallowfield has interviewed many breast cancer patients about their feelings, and she has found that women commonly feel cancer is their punishment for past 'bad' (i.e. sexual) behaviour:

> When I found the lump I knew exactly what it was and I thought this is my punishment at last for what I did. You see, I had an illegitimate baby when I was nineteen and I kept her. You didn't do things like that in my day, although it seems all right to be an unmarried mother nowadays. Anyway, I've always lied and told everyone that my husband was dead.

> This is God's punishment for my wickedness. I had an affair once with a married man. I'd always had large breasts and that's what attracted him, I suppose.

Long buried in our thinking then, are some complex and difficult associations with breasts. On the one hand, breasts mean pleasure, beauty, comfort, nurture. But on the other, they mean shame, discomfort, failure, death.

The taboos surrounding breasts have been strong enough to stop previous generations from discussing them seriously, and from exposing the damaging myths. They also seem to have prevented serious research into breasts. One of the most startling facts to emerge from this book's research is the almost total lack of any study into breasts except by scientists concerned with cancer.

We need to know more about breasts if we are to understand the taboos and confront the myths. We need to talk about breasts – with our friends, with our lovers, with our daughters – if we are to break the chain which links breasts to 'sin', if we are to regain pleasure, pride and a sense of control over our own bodies.

2
Breasts and men

So why *are* men – at least, Western men – so fixated by breasts? I've tried asking them, without much success. It's not something most men have thought much about; they take it for granted as 'natural'. It's not something (or so I'm told) they discuss among themselves, except in macho mode. Nor have the 'experts' looked into the subject: I could find no published research in the psychosexual field which explores attitudes to breasts. The only studies available deal solely with mastectomy.

Yet on one level it's easy to find out what men feel about breasts. This is a male-dominated society, and we are surrounded by images of breasts, comments on breasts, stories, books, films, magazines, jokes and pornography about breasts. In this culture, breasts are everywhere – but nowhere. In trying to understand male attitudes to breasts it's hard to see the wood for the trees.

This chapter sets out to explore the strange wood which is Western man's obsession with breasts.

Breasts around the world

Although it's hard to believe, for anyone who has grown up in Britain, breasts are not a universal sex symbol. Men from countries with different cultural traditions are not so fixated by breasts and find our attitudes ridiculous.

In Japan – where the women have comparatively small breasts – the back of the neck is reputedly an area of intense erotic interest. I am told that napes appear in Japanese pornography much as breasts appear in Western pornography. The Maori people, according to Naomi Wolf in *The Beauty Myth*, think a fat vulva is the ultimate in female allure.

Many African societies take a very relaxed attitude to breasts too, concentrating on a woman's thighs and bottom as the area of maximum eroticism. The writer Gabrielle Palmer, who has lived in Mozambique, says that urban Mozambican women will go to work in Westernized clothes, but when they get home they change for comfort into a 'cloth' – which is worn around the waist, leaving the breasts bare. She has sat in Mozambican cinemas where people have not reacted at all to breasts revealed in love scenes. But as soon as a bottom is revealed, a gasp goes up from the entire audience:

> Showing your flanks is very sexual in African society. The haunches are a sexual symbol. Some women have a tattoo on their thigh which they will only allow a lover to see. I have a friend from Uganda, and although she is a sophisticated woman, she still gets embarrassed when she sees Western women wearing shorts in hot weather.

Yet, says Gabrielle Palmer, breasts can be bared – even touched – in African society, without too much excitement:

I've watched an African man flirting with a woman he is clearly planning to go to bed with. Yet she has a baby on her back and one bare breast hanging down. He is not fetishizing that part of her body, or going berserk about it as a Western man would. I've also known an African man to touch a woman friend's breast, and she was able to tell me quite categorically that it was not a sexual gesture. Contrast that to the situation in America where a 'lactation consultant' (a private practitioner who helps mothers with breast-feeding problems) has to be very careful not to touch a mother's breast as she positions the baby – because she can be sued for sexual assault.

Bug-eyed Westerners . . .

In the Gambia too, say Western aid workers, young girls work bare-breasted. But should a Westerner arrive, those same girls will cover their breasts – because they know Westerners are upset by breasts. And in Papua New Guinea, a woman who falls over so that her grass skirt lifts up and reveals her genitals is said to experience such shame that she may commit suicide. Yet she comfortably walks around bare-breasted.

There is a certain comedy value in stories of bug-eyed Western men plunged into cultures where breasts are bared all around them. According to a teacher who once worked in Africa (his wife told me this story), the young women of the village where he lived went about topless as a matter of course. These women only covered their breasts when first married. As soon as they became mothers, their breasts were bared again. At first, this Western man found all those young, bare breasts a riveting sight as he shopped at the market or walked to work. But as time went by, he found that he lost his initial sense of excitement and began to take bare breasts for granted.

Western culture has not always been so concerned with breasts. During the early Middle Ages, the rounded belly was deliberately emphasized. Elizabethan women, too, dressed so that their breasts were available to babies, and says Gabrielle Palmer, lactation was seen as integral to a woman's sexual attractiveness.

More recently, in the 1920s, 'flappers' bound their breasts to make them appear non-existent. And in the sixties, legs temporarily took over as the focus of erotic attention. Perhaps change is in the air yet again: Paul Brown, a consulting clinical psychiatrist and founding member of the Association of Sexual and Marital Therapy, has noticed that the female crotch now seems to be an alternative area of intense sexual interest.

No longer mummy's boy

There is a maxim that every man born has had to fight his way out from under the domination of a woman. Certainly, it is a great insult in our culture to call a man a 'mummy's boy'. Males have to make the break from the first person they have loved – their mother – and they are expected to make it early.

Paul Brown believes that our culture's early separation of male from female sets up terrific problems for men later in life. Many of his patients are men who have been sent to public school, a small but highly influential group:

Many men who come to see me are uncovering the incredible pain of their early childhood experiences, in particular the pain of being sent away from their mothers at an early age. This leaves a desperate longing which they spend their lives trying to fill.

Breasts are symbolic of that lost maternal love, and so they become objects of intense desire. However, they are also associated with fear because they remind men of that early experience of rejection. As a result, many men are in the grip of intense, conflicting (and often buried) love/hate feelings towards breasts, and these feelings fuel our culture's breast obsessions.

According to Tom Ryan, a psychotherapist writing in *The Sexuality of Men*, many men fear closeness and intimacy with women because of women's 'overwhelming powers'. These men distance themselves from women in various ways in order to feel in continuous control. Ryan describes the case of 'Dave', a man who came for therapy because of his inability to commit himself to a relationship without feeling anxious and fearful. Dave was considered a 'sissy' (synonymous with 'mummy's boy') by his father and his brother because of his close relationship with his mother:

Dave is attracted, for what at first seem to be aesthetic reasons, to women of 'angular and athletic' build. He wishes his partners to be 'firm and sharp'. In other words, there must be no hint of softness or largeness, particularly in the breasts – what Dave calls the 'motherly type'. On occasions when Dave has seen or been with a 'fat' or 'large' woman, he experiences a sensation of being lost or enveloped by their 'layers of flesh'. I believe what Dave fears most is his own wish to be enveloped, to be lost in the woman. A fear and a wish exist simultaneously.

Murdering mammaries!

Suffocation by breasts is a recurrent male fantasy. (There is a related myth that babies can be suffocated by breastfeeding – see Chapter Four.) In the 1986 James Bond film *The Living Daylights* a man is killed by being crushed to death between a woman's breasts. In a Hollywood film by breast-obsessed Russ Meyer, called *Chesty Morgan and Her Deadly Weapons*, men are again the victims of murdering mammaries.

But behind these fears of being dominated or suffocated by women is the desire to be like a woman, to surrender to her and to be united with her. Tom Ryan believes our culture's preoccupation with male cross-dressing, even at the level of panto dames and men in drag for fancy-dress parties, is a sign of how insecure men are in their sexual identity and how they sometimes yearn to be a woman. The man with a handbag and two balloons stuffed under his jumper is a familiar figure in British comedy. Perhaps we should be thinking less in terms of 'penis envy' when it comes to relationships between the sexes, and more in terms of 'breast envy'.

The intense and contradictory feelings conjured by breasts are not a modern phenomenon. In her book *Monuments and Maidens*, the cultural historian Marina Warner points out that in the *Iliad*, Hecuba exposes her breast to her son Hector, imploring him not to go into battle against Achilles.

'Hector, my child,' she cries, opening her dress to hold her breast towards him, 'have some regard for this and pity me. How often have I given you this breast and soothed you with its milk! Bear in mind those days, dear child.' This appeal to be loyal to the private, maternal world of love and intimacy is rejected by Hector. He chooses instead the public, masculine role of warrior and goes out to battle – and to death.

In Aeschylus' *Oresteia*, Clytemnestra, mother of Orestes, makes a similar appeal. This time, the purpose is to stop Orestes from murdering her – she whose breasts sustained him and gave him life.

'Wait son,' says Clytemnestra, 'no feeling for this, my child? The breast you held, drowsing away the hours, soft gums tugging the milk that made you grow?'

For a moment, Orestes seems to waver. But his mother's breast reminds him of deeper conflicts too, reminds him that she is sexual as well as maternal and that she has had sex with a man who was not his father. He kills her.

In these stories the breast symbolizes motherhood and love: these are precious necessities without which the human race could not survive. But it also suggests sex and female power, forces which men have long feared.

Beautiful is big

One of the reasons why our society is so ambivalent about breasts is tied up with our attitudes to beauty. By and large, we are not a nation that values the aesthetically beautiful. Paul Brown argues that we suffer a deep cultural impoverishment which shows itself in a middle-class male contempt for all art forms and a suspicion that male artists (ballet dancers, opera singers, painters) are likely to be 'poofters' or 'sissies':

> In contrast to the Continent where people have an appreciation of beauty, British men have not been taught to value the beautiful or the attractive. It is all degraded to a matter of size. Many women

will apologize for their small breast size at the beginning of a relationship, because size is the only dimension they see as being valued.

Breast deprivation

We are the third generation of a society which has largely given up breastfeeding in favour of bottle-feeding. However in the past, human beings have always suckled infants at the breast (not always at the mother's breast, but at breasts none the less). That early relation between woman and child was automatic and unquestionable, creating the foundations for mental, emotional and physical health throughout human history.

Every woman who has ever fed a baby knows the overpowering need of her baby for the breast (as well as her own strong urge to feed her baby). What have we done in abandoning that natural pattern and choosing an artificial, lifeless substitute for the breast? The implications for adult life (not to mention infant life) are staggering, yet they have never been properly researched.

Adult sexual life – and so men's attitudes to breasts – is connected to our babyhood experiences, as Andy Metcalf, writing in *The Sexuality of Men*, explains:

> Sex for both men and women carries many more meanings than an erotic impulse. Through skin-to-skin contact, stroking and caressing, it mimics early infant life and can reinvoke powerful levels of well-being. In its symbolic recreation of our infant existence, sexual activity may become the vehicle for a number of conflicting emotions: love, hostility or dependency.

Therefore, the absence of breasts in our infant experiences

must have a bearing on this generation's sexuality and on all the feelings that go with it. Andrea Whalley, former director of Breast Cancer Care, is quite clear that our mass defection to bottle-feeding is behind modern man's obsession with breasts:

> It's the bottle which is to blame, I'm sure of it. Men haven't had enough suckling at the breast when they were babies.

Gabrielle Palmer points to the amount of pornography that focusses on the sucking of the breast:

> It's extraordinary that grown men of our culture are so obsessed with suckling. You have to ask – were those men deprived as children? The attitude that 'those breasts belong to me', however, is very Western. I cannot imagine men of other cultures being jealous of their child being breastfed.

Battleground of the sex war

We are also living in a time of rapid social change, particularly in the roles of the sexes. We have abandoned many of the traditional Western markers that make it obvious that a woman is a woman, such as skirts, lipstick and long hair. In these unisex decades, many women wear jeans and T-shirts, like men. They go out to work, like men. They can look very much like men – except that they have breasts.

Breasts remain the one, indisputable outward sign that a woman is a woman. As a result, breasts have become more important in how we perceive people. Men – and women too – have become more conscious of breasts as a sign of sexual identity. It's a short step from there to see how breasts have been elevated into symbols of womanhood, of sex, of difference. This is how breasts have become a battleground in today's sex war.

For decades women have been claiming that there is more to life than our biological role. Yet the emphasis on breasts is a constant reminder of this role. Bare breasts, vulnerable breasts – on display everywhere – are seen by women as a statement that some men prefer to see us as the decorative sex, the passive, to-be-looked-at sex, the bearers of 'boobs', 'jubblies', 'titties', the to-be-ridiculed sex.

It's not surprising then if women feel the male obsession with breasts is an extended put-down, an ongoing act of revenge for women's attempts to assert their freedom from traditional roles. What does at first seem surprising is that so few male partners of 'liberated' women seem to understand or respect that view. Or do they secretly relish the put-down that lies behind the pin-up?

Getting to grips with breasts

In the meantime, modern Western men have quite a problem. How do they behave when confronted with breasts? The short answer – which is the answer men tend to give – is sexually. As one man told his wife when she questioned him:

> I like them very much. I like to touch them, hold them, look at them.

But what do men do about all those more complex, more contradictory feelings they have for breasts? What do they do about breasts as a symbol of all they want and all they fear? How do they preserve the façade of manly control in the face of this powerful, threatening, desired object?

If men can separate breasts from individual women, objectify them, make jokes about them or vilify them, then they have progressed a long way towards being able to control their fear of female power, their fear of maternal influence.

The jokes are legion, from the schoolyard 'have you seen my Titswobble?' number, to the Carry On/Benny Hill/Ronnie Barker/seaside postcard variety and the endless throwaway lines of the stand-up comedian ('I've seen bigger lumps in oatmeal'). The best gag in the world, they say, is 'tits'. Men love to laugh about breasts: laughter defuses the tension around sexuality and puts them back in control.

Richard Dyer, a counsellor writing in *The Sexuality of Men*, argues that although the butt of sexual comedy often seems to be a woman, the joke is often really about men. While acknowledging that much male humour takes a derogatory and spiteful view of women, he believes the 'busty blonde' type of comedy is particularly concerned with exposing male weakness:

> Comedy turns terror into laughter ... But [it also] expresses male fears and anxieties about female sexual energy, about the way it may test virility, about the way it challenges male supremacy.
>
> Jayne Mansfield, Barbara Windsor and the string of performers featured in Benny Hill's shows are often at the centre of gags concerned with the extraordinary impact on men of overwhelming, uncontrollable sexual arousal. When Mansfield walks down the street in *The Girl Can't Help It*, a man unloading a huge block of ice finds it turning to steam in his hands – her impact just turns him red hot ... Many Benny Hill sketches are simply built around him starting off doing something and being instantly, ineluctably, catastrophically, but delightedly distracted by a bouncily-bosomed

blonde woman walking by. Benny Hill in pursuit of women is never anything other than foolish to look at.

Laughing and gawping at the breasts of women 'out there' – women in films, saucy postcards and pin-ups – can also help men to ignore the fact that the real women in their lives are so emotionally powerful. After all, if a man is going to be a 'failure' in his manhood – i.e. his heterosexuality – a woman is going to be the first person to know about it.

If men can think of breasts as 'out there', as separate from an individual, they can enjoy looking at breasts without having to have a relationship with the person behind the breasts:

> My husband will spend hours on the sofa watching Continental movies – just for the chance of a glimpse of someone else's breast. I have said to him on occasion – here you are, have a look at mine if you like – but he says I'm missing the point, as it were.

It is as if the topless image becomes a kind of talisman against men's fear of women's sexuality. The women who pose with bare breasts, whether on page three or in men's magazines, always turn their gaze invitingly on the male viewer, giving him the message that he is desirable. In looking at pin-ups a man can safely deal with breasts, he can look without risk at what threatens to 'unman' him. He is made powerful. Breasts are made manageable.

'Unfulfilled appetites, ancient confusions'

The American writer Philip Roth has tried to tackle the male dilemma over breasts in his blackly humorous novel *The Breast*. Roth's 'hero' is David Kepesh, a highly cerebral lecturer in literature at an American university, who discovers he has been metamorphosed into a six-foot-long breast overnight.

In trying to make sense of his monstrous, Kafkaesque transformation, Kepesh remembers his girlfriend Claire's breast being lowered into his mouth during lovemaking 'as though it were the globe itself – soft globe! – and I some Poseidon or Zeus!' At the time, Kepesh had experienced 'breast envy' (the novel substitutes 'breast' for 'penis' in a number of ways), and he has felt the desire 'to be breasted, or to be Claire's breast'.

Later, Kepesh asks himself why this happened:

> Why was it a breast I had imagined myself to be? What whirling chaos of desire and fear had erupted in this primitive identification with the object of infantile veneration? What unfulfilled appetites or ancient confusions, what fragments of my remotest past could have collided?

Was it a teenage diet too rich in centrefolds, he wonders, or was it the male longing to be female, to be other, which caused his catastrophe?

> Was it a longing . . . to be utterly and blessedly helpless, to be a big, brainless bag of tissue, desirable, dumb, passive, immobile, acted upon instead of acting . . . Or think of it as some form of hibernation, a long winter's sleep buried in the mountains of the female anatomy. Or think of the breast as my cocoon, first cousin to that sac in which I trod my mother's waters.

The breast means oblivion, chaos, loss of male individuality. It is the enemy and the opposite of the phallic – which is distinct, directed, active, goal-oriented.

Kepesh desperately seeks to remember his first breastfeeding experiences:

> I dredge the muck of my beginnings in search of a single glittering memory of my hungering gums at the spigot, my nose in the nourishing globe.

But the poor man cannot get a grip. His rational faculties are no match for his primeval, instinctual origins:

> It is all too far back, back where I am. I claw the slime at the sea bottom, but by the time I rise to the surface there is not even silt beneath my fingernails.

Kepesh's lapse into identification with the female, his uncontrolled desire for the breast, has betrayed him. He has submitted to the mammary, he has returned to the helplessness of babyhood. He is unmanned.

Not in front of the boys

Of course, men aren't supposed to admit to such anxieties. In public – especially in the company of other men – they tend to adopt jocular or macho attitudes. Raise the subject of breasts in a group of men and the grins are instant, the jokes and puns only seconds away. Chances are that they will start cupping their hands, drawing curvy shapes in the air and making grunting, growling noises. An important male bonding ritual is under way and women are excluded by the laughter. Unlike women, says Paul Brown:

Men generally don't talk intimately. When they do talk, it tends to be a kind of locker-room talk which is about 'scoring'. In English male society it is extremely terrifying to talk about feelings, as a man is likely to be laughed at. There is an English cult that it is bad for mothers to allow boys to have feelings as, if they have feelings, there is a risk that they will turn into homosexuals.

Deep feelings about sex are kept particularly quiet, believes Andy Metcalf:

These days sex is a fraught affair for many men. It is a topic we break away from or parry with a joke. There is a silence about it; in all the voluminous literature about sex and sexuality, there is very little on male sexuality as such. Most of the men contributing to this book [*The Sexuality of Men*] have discovered that it is also a hidden subject, resistant to their first investigations. It seems as if it's so much an accepted part of life that it is invisible . . . Beneath the macho posing and the bedroom performance, many men have unsure and conflicting feelings about their sexuality.

When men do communicate intimately it tends to be with their women partners – and many women have told me that their man's private attitudes to breasts are quite different from the public stance:

In keeping with a long-established sexual double standard (there is the kind of girl men want to sleep with versus the kind they want to marry), there are the breasts men like to gawp at versus the breasts they want to go home to at night.

What men like to look at 'out there' is completely different from what men like in bed with them.

I think men are conditioned to think that 'big boobs' are supposed to be sexy, and that they are supposed to 'nudge nudge, wink wink' when they are with their male friends. But in fact, in private, their own preferences can be entirely different when it comes to the real thing.

I think men are very frightened of women's sexuality. Women are very much part of the forces of nature. And as Camille Paglia has pointed out, we have all these secrets. Our sexual organs can't be seen. A man can't tell if it's his child that is being carried by a pregnant woman, or not. There are all these things that men will never know about women, and it bothers them. Breasts are symbolic of all that.

I think men are terrified of breasts.

In an article in American *Cosmopolitan*, writer Eric Pooley came out of the closet about breasts:

There is a difference between the urban male's public behaviour and his private thoughts. The public carryings-on, especially when he is travelling with a pack, may be offhandedly boorish and crude, left over from the Pleistocene Age. The private thoughts may also be pre-historic – but just as probable, they are thoroughly modern and reflect an expansive vision of beauty with plenty of room for all sorts of physical types, from voluptuous to what's sometimes called boyish. A vision that grows and changes with time. One that's far from anything dreamed of at seventeen.

When men congregate, a lot of us have trouble admitting to anything that seems remotely enlightened. (It's just so much fun to be a howling jerk.) But the enlightened attitudes are there. Get a man alone and maybe you'll see them emerge, cautiously.

Most women know that when men fall in love with them,

they fall in love with the whole person, not with her breasts (or legs, or bum . . .). Generally speaking, men seem to love the body parts belonging to the women they love – not to choose a woman on the basis of her body parts (although they *may* be strongly attractive elements at the beginning).

Most women also seem quite secure about their own man's private feelings for their breasts. In a survey by Drs Andrew and Penny Stanway (*The Breast*), half said their partners were 'highly satisfied', and a quarter thought their partners were 'fairly satisfied' with their breasts. Only 15 per cent thought their partners would alter their breasts if they could.

Sniggering

It's doubly irritating for women who know men's private sensibilities, who know they have a real, erotic and appreciative relationship with their breasts, to witness them acting like 'howling jerks':

> It's his sniggering at other women's breasts which I find very upsetting. We went on holiday to a place with topless beaches, and apparently it amazes him that all women's breasts are different. It amazes me that he's amazed. After all, our faces are not all the same, so why should our breasts be? And his behaviour makes me feel belittled. I would like to be able to strip off on the beach too, but I don't want to be compared – positively or negatively – with other women. I am quite happy with my breasts. They should be treated as just another part of my body.

The worst of the sniggering, of course, comes in tabloid form, and the bigger the breasts, the bigger the snigger. 'Pandora Peaks', who reputedly has a bust measurement of 62HHH, has been a favourite of the *Sun* newspaper. The *Sun* went to town on Pandora in her custom-made, steel-reinforced bras, referring to her 'TIN PEAKS' and 'H-H-HUGE ASSETS'.

Russ Meyer told the *Sun* (30.9.92), 'She's got the greatest t*ts in the world. We're talking big bazookas here.' The *Sun* described the reaction from 'hordes of slobbering men' as Pandora danced in a club:

> When Pandora struts her stuff – in gangster, nurse and cowboy outfits – tongues are on the floor . . . 'Where the hell did she get a pair like that?' [remarks one punter]. 'Half the guys in town are here because I guess it's as much of a freak show as a turn on.'

The first thought of any woman who sees a picture of Pandora is – how *painful* it must be to have breasts that big. To their credit, the *Sun* sent a woman journalist to ask Pandora about the physical realities of her shape (9.10.92). In a story entitled LIFE IS HELL WITH MORE THAN YOUR PAIR SHARE, it was revealed that Pandora can't live a normal life. She can't even walk normally. She can only hobble along slowly, and running is impossible for her.

Nor can Pandora sleep easily. Lying on her front is out of the question and even lying on her side is uncomfortable. She has to wear a special sleep bra. During the day she has to keep her back ramrod straight at all times to support her breasts, and if she makes any quick movements she suffers twinges of pain. (But on the same page the *Sun* printed a picture of smiling Pandora, her vast bra overflowing with £1 coins: 'Win the contents of Pandora's bra! Everyone wants to get their hands on Pandora's assets! Call 0839 . . .')

Surviving the breast blitz

Various studies have been done on the effects of porn on men, but has anybody ever seriously asked about the effects of pin-ups on women? By suggesting that the atypical Pandora shape – or simply the firm teenage shape of many pin-ups – is the admired one, women with 'normal' breasts are given the message that their breasts are inferior. As this woman in her thirties put it:

> I think you have to be very confident in your own body, and believe strongly that you have the right to be loved as you are, not to feel influenced by the barrage of images of so-called bodily perfection everywhere you turn.

Certainly, the MP Clare Short received thousands of supporting letters from women when she tried to get Parliament to ban page-three girls in the tabloids. Some women linked their own experiences of sexual assault to the topless images. Women who had experienced rape described how their male attackers compared them to page-three girls in the course of the rape, or said, 'You should be on page three.'

Other women said they felt put down by being constantly compared with and contrasted to the page-three 'lovelies'. One woman who had had a mastectomy for breast cancer wrote of her pain and humiliation as her husband brought page-three pictures into the house day after day. Teachers described how children reacted when tabloid newspapers were used for school artwork: as soon as they saw the bare breasts of the pin-ups, little boys began to snigger and little girls stood about embarrassed, not knowing what to do.

Phoney fantasy

Bare breasts aren't confined to the tabloids. They turn up everywhere from clubs to pubs to workplaces. And because the models either have that soppy 'come-hither' message in their eyes, or the corny 'dying-for-it' look, the topless image constantly promotes a phoney male fantasy of relationships with women.

Perhaps it wouldn't be so bad if we saw topless women with expressions of irony, of intelligence – even of boredom – on their faces. At least we would know they had some identity, some individuality. It's the anodyne 'nice girl next door' image which is so irritating to other women. The bare breasts themselves are often beautiful: it's the paid-for, male-adoring expressions on the faces which are so dishonest.

But what can women do under the 'breast blitz'? Ignoring pin-ups implies a kind of acceptance: it's 'harmless fun' for men to depict women this way. Of course we all know that breasts are fun in the bedroom, but when we are trying to do our jobs or get the car fixed, pin-ups can only serve as a statement of male control.

Taking action to get rid of pin-ups, on the other hand, can take perseverance, at the very least. This woman did try, gently and humorously at first, but unsuccessfully. Having given up, she was left with a nasty sense of collusion:

> For ten years I've worked in a workshop (at my husband's business) that has been plastered with pictures of nude women. In the past I have drawn felt-pen underwear on them, but I gave up, because frankly there weren't enough hours in the day to cover up all these pictures.
>
> But now, for the first time, my fifteen-year-old son is working in the workshop during the holidays. Before he went there I made my

husband take down every single picture. I can live with the thought of my husband being surrounded by them, but I cannot live with the idea of my son having to do the same. He is too young. If he has seen this stuff it has been 'out there'. It hasn't come into his home.

I am protecting his psyche, and mine. I don't want him to feel that his father or I have sanctioned those pictures. Although it's true they have been sanctioned up till now. We are all the more principled when it comes to our children. I hope there's a picture of Nora Batty up there instead: now she's a real woman!

Up front about breasts

Slowly, things are changing. By the early 1990s the page-three image was losing its glamour. Page-three models were losing their celebrity status – and their huge incomes – to the new supermodels. There were even rumours that the *Sun* was thinking of dropping the page, although at the time of writing it is still going strong.

Certainly this generation is likely to be more relaxed about breasts than the men who grew up with their sexuality seared by the huge and thrusting 1950s Hollywood bosom. These days women's shapes in film and fashion are more various and more natural. True, models are under pressure to have breast implants, but the nude bodies (still always female) of television drama and film are not uniformly voluptuous.

This generation has travelled more, too, and come into contact with different attitudes in different cultures. Even the topless beaches of overseas holiday resorts have their educational value.

As this man in his thirties wrote in response to my questionnaire:

> I think a lot of attention is drawn to breasts by the social norm of hiding them. On a nudist beach, for instance, nobody takes much notice. [He is a man who also described himself as 'very pleased' that his child was breastfed.]

Older women have said to me that they think the young men of today are more open about a range of sexual and emotional issues. The emotional barriers that have isolated men in the past may not yet have broken down, but at least more men are aware of them.

Today's women are more likely to demand honesty, self-knowledge and communication from their menfolk. They are more likely to challenge their men about porn and pin-ups too, and to insist that women are treated with respect. Breast disease has also ceased to be an unmentionable subject.

We can hope that as the sex roles change, the sharp traditional divides between mothers (sole carers of children) and fathers (emotionally distant) will continue to soften. If so, there is a good chance that future men will be less fearful of the 'mummy's boy' label, less divided in themselves about women and about their sexuality – and less gripped by obsessive love/hate feelings towards breasts.

3
Beauty and the breast

Breasts are vital to a woman's sense of her own attractiveness and femininity. And contrary to a common assumption that all women complain about their bodies, most women who have talked to me in the course of this book have said that they like their breasts. Some have even said they think their breasts are the most beautiful aspects of themselves.

Sadly, there are also many women whose lives are made miserable by the belief that their breasts are 'ugly' or somehow 'wrong'. Either they have grown up with insecurities about their breasts, comparing themselves unfavourably with the fantasy breasts of Hollywood stars and pin-ups, or they have come to fear male criticism that their breasts are 'too big', 'too small' or in the 'wrong shape'.

This chapter turns criticism back onto the everchanging standards of beauty itself, and looks at how the fashion industry and the media influence those standards.

It also looks at the lengths women will go to in order not to 'fail' in attractiveness and femininity. One way of 'improving' beauty is to have cosmetic breast surgery. Here, two women who have had their breast size changed explain why they did it and what it was like, while a breast surgeon adds her point of view.

'He bought me cornplasters and said – these should fit you . . .'

Jenny is twenty-seven, and she told me about her breast implants seven months after her NHS operation:

I never liked my breasts. They were too small: I was 32A on one side, and 30 A A on the other. It had bothered me since I was about sixteen. I was the only one at school not wearing a bra.

I was teased, mostly by my family. My brothers kept saying, 'How come you haven't developed yet?' And on my eighteenth birthday my dad bought me some cornplasters and said, 'I didn't know your bra size, but these should fit.'

It was spoiling my life, because of the way I saw myself. I went through a lot of mental pain and trouble. I wouldn't go out. I wouldn't do anything. I couldn't wear feminine clothes. I felt in limbo about my sexuality. When I looked in the mirror I felt more of a man than a woman, although I've got two children.

I was affected by outside influences – like the media. Those pressures are wrong, but they're real. And I think most men want a woman to have a pair of breasts.

I breastfed my first baby for two weeks, and my second for two months. I thought my breasts were too small and that I never had enough milk. It was trial and error, really. I had no support from anyone in breastfeeding – so I stuck them both on the bottle after a while.

It was my second child who ruined my breasts. At least they were the same size before she was born, but then one got even smaller and shrivelled up.

A couple of years ago a friend bought me a basque. It was the smallest size he could get, but when I put it on I thought 'aaargh!'. He showed me a book with information about breast implants. I had thought that was only for the page-three type, not for the likes of me. But the book said it was the second most common form of cosmetic surgery in America (after the nose job).

When I went to see my doctor I was really nervous and worried. I was too embarrassed to tell a man what I wanted to do, so I saw the nurse first and asked her to speak to the doctor for me. I was also afraid it would be too expensive for me. When I saw the doctor I was crying and shaking. I was a bag of nerves. He kept passing me tissues and he said he would arrange for me to see the specialist in nineteen weeks' time.

When I saw the specialist I had to take my T-shirt off in front of him. It was very embarrassing. I thought, 'oh no, I don't want this', and I was crying again.

He had a look at me and said, 'Yes, that's fine. You've got a problem, we can sort you out.' He said he could put implants under the muscle on my chest. He also said if I had the operation I couldn't have any more kids, so I decided to be sterilized at the same time. I didn't ask any questions at the time, and he didn't tell me about any risks. I just wanted it done.

Soon after I saw a television programme about a woman who had been partially paralysed when her foam implant leaked into her body. That worried me. But I went into Frenchay Hospital in Bristol. The specialist said there was no need for me to be sterilized, that I could still have kids after the implant. That was a relief. But for nearly a year I had worked myself up to the idea of no more children unnecessarily.

They took a photograph of my body before the operation. It was a male photographer, although they apologized and said it was usually a woman. I had to take my T-shirt off and stand up – very embarrassing.

I got most of my information on the night before the operation. But I found it hard to remember my questions, as well as the answers. The nurses were really helpful. I wanted to know if I was going to be paralysed like the woman on the television programme. I asked them about all my fears.

One doctor came to talk to me and said there was no guarantee. It was always possible that implants could break – although being gel they would blob out rather than leak out. He also said that the scar tissue around the implant could be hard. The implants could only last about ten years, after which I may need another operation.

He told me I would have to be careful for six weeks – I mustn't even lift my arms to wash my hair or pick up the milk. He went through all the bad things, but then he said that thousands of women have had it done and they are quite okay.

So I thought – well, you only live once. I am going to have it done. I told a few friends and they said, 'We never noticed you were particularly small.' I said, 'That's all the big T-shirts I've been wearing.'

It was very strange when I woke up. I felt huge. I thought – what have they done! I didn't want them *this* big! I felt quite excited, but shocked as well. I had been turned into a 34B. I'm now a 36B because I'm pregnant again.

I had a tubigrip bandage on with drains for the first three days, but I could see my new outline. When they took it off (I had a shot of morphine as they took the drains out) I looked at them and thought, 'Now, this is alright!' I liked them straight away. I was beaming, really pleased. All the doctors were having a look too, but I didn't mind: I had something to look at, at last.

The scars underneath my breasts were quite long – about three inches – and half-an-inch wide. The cuts were stuck together without stitches, so as not to leave marks. I wasn't too pleased about them, but they won't stay for ever. I can also use scar cover make-up. There was pain, but I was expecting that and I knew it wouldn't last. There was discomfort and a strangeness for about four weeks while the muscle grew back. Now, nine months later, one nipple is still a bit numb from time to time. The other one is just as before. The implants are quite soft. I like my new body.

My brothers asked me why I had it done, and I said, 'I'd had enough of you lot taking the mickey.' They apologized to me then.

It's been wonderful. It has changed my life. I don't worry about going out now. I can wear what I want. I can go swimming and to aerobics. The paranoia is gone: I've got confidence. I can be like a woman.

'I was known as "the biggest boobs in town" . . .'

Lesley works as a hairdresser. She is married with two children, and she told me about her breast reduction seven months after her NHS operation:

My size didn't worry me too much while I was at school. I was quite happy with myself, although I was known to be a bit 'booby'.

But I must have been naïve, because a few years later a friend of mine met one of our old teachers. He said, 'How's your friend? I can't remember her name: the one with the big boobs . . .' It stemmed from that really. It was such a shock to realize how they looked at me, how they remembered me.

You learn to dress accordingly, in baggy tops, nothing high-necked (it makes you look larger), and I always wore bras which were too small so that they would squash me. Buying dresses was difficult: I was a size 12 at the waist, and a size 20 on top. My bras had thick straps, but they only lasted a couple of months. The elastic would ride high up my back and I was always trying to hoik it down.

I'm a hairdresser and someone once told me that men loved it when I washed their hair. I resented that. I was only doing my job. And there was a man who used to say to me, 'Here's the lady with the biggest boobs in town.' If a man had got a very big nose, I wouldn't make remarks about that. I never used to react, but everything they said registered with me. The remarks just went in and sort of hovered inside.

As a woman you can never relax about your body. When we go swimming we are always tucking bits in, and shielding other bits. Men don't have to do that. It's the media which makes us self-conscious. I hate page three. It makes me angry, what they portray about women.

And then I had real problems when I got pregnant. I was at least an F-cup, and I went into Mothercare to enquire about feeding bras. They had never had anyone asking for a bra at my size. So I went on to an old-fashioned corsetry shop, but they also said there was nothing they could do for me. Eventually I contacted the NCT and got the biggest bra size they had.

Breastfeeding was very difficult being so large. I had to support my breast with my hand as well as supporting the baby. I got back trouble and was very uncomfortable. It was difficult to find clothes for myself. I weaned the baby at six weeks and prayed my breasts would shrink, but they didn't. They were horrendous: droopy, stretched, and long with furrows and marks down them.

I did go to aerobics and I got really fit and thin – except for my saggy breasts. I'd wear four layers at aerobics to hold me: a bra, crop top, leotard, and another top.

My mum first suggested I see a doctor. I was quite shocked! My husband and I both had our worries about surgery, but he thought that if it made me happy it was a good thing. But when I did go to my GP I got quite upset. He accepted the idea of surgery straight away and said he could refer me to a specialist. That was awful: I had to take my top off and sit there, feeling very self-conscious. He told me what he could do for me, but I didn't really take it in. I wasn't looking for perfect, I was looking for smaller. The waiting list was at least a year.

When my second baby was seven weeks old I went back to the specialist. My milk had gone, but I was large. They took photographs of my body, which was very embarrassing. But they were wonderful at the hospital. I told them I was really worried and they went through all the details with me.

I had it done two weeks later. I was on an NHS plastic surgery ward. There were elderly people having skin grafts, and there was I having my 'boobs' done. I felt very guilty; I didn't 'need' this. But the nurses were wonderful. I expected them to say, 'Oh, you are silly', but they didn't.

The doctor drew all over my chest with a bright blue pen. I was in the operating theatre and recovery for three-and-a-half hours altogether. They took three-quarters of a pound from one breast, one pound from another – the equivalent of four apples from one and three from the other. I wondered what they did with my flesh: did they give it to someone else who wanted to be bigger? They made a horseshoe-shaped cut beneath my breasts, cut straight up to the nipple, and all around the nipple, which they then moved up.

I wasn't with it for a day or two, and then I was uncomfortable but not in pain. I was all bandaged up with a drain in each side – which was horrible. When they took the bandages off the surgeon tickled my nipples, and they were really sensitive. Two weeks later my breasts looked fantastic, no bruising, and that was it, no need to go back. It was like a fairy tale. I couldn't believe it.

They say you can't expect to breastfeed after the operation, although some women do. They had also warned me that I wouldn't have much sensation in my nipples, although there wasn't much before. I do have some feeling in my nipples, although they are quite numbed. I don't consider it a problem. Yes, I've got scars but they're not bad – the worst are under my arms, not on my breasts.

My family were all very pleased. I asked my mum what my dad thought and she said, 'He thinks you should be happy with what God's given you, but if it makes you happier, well and good.'

But even though they were a lovely shape (I'm a B-cup now), I've only just accepted them as *me* – after seven months. They were so different. It's like when you get your hair cut. You need time to come to terms.

My husband does prefer them this way. I've said to him, 'You're lucky, you've had the choice of two types of breasts on the same woman.' Other people who know about it have said how brave I was. But generally people just think I've lost weight.

I can now wear dresses I would never have dreamed of wearing before. And I'm looking forward to this summer and going swimming. I've still got to get out of the habit of putting my hands in front of me when I run. I've been to aerobics without so much as a sports bra, and I was fine. It's been wonderful. It has changed my life.

Now my mum wants to have it done. She's sixty-three. She hasn't told my dad yet: I don't know what he will say. But she has been to her doctor. I thought, good for you mum!

'It's a dramatic change'

Ruth Lester, FRCS, is a consultant plastic surgeon in Birmingham,
with both NHS and private patients. Breast implants are a significant
proportion of her work:

At first, I must admit, I found it difficult to understand why
women wanted to have implants. But now I have seen so
many women so happy after having them. Some are so
upset by their own body image. They are aware of the risks
involved, but are prepared to take them.

I know that people's quality of life is improved by augmentation. It's a matter of self-image. Ladies with very small
breasts don't feel feminine. For them, going swimming or
undressing in front of a partner becomes a nightmare. With
implants they become more confident. It's a dramatic
change. They come back and say things like, 'I've gone on
stage for the first time', or, 'my relationship has improved'.
They're happier. It's very satisfying.

I explain all the possible complications to patients. Yes, if
you put an implant in you are going against nature and
putting yourself slightly at risk. But women have to make up
their own minds. Is their quality of life likely to be so
improved that they will take a slight risk? I compare it to the
risks of driving down the motorway, or flying – a very small
risk.

I'm sure women have been influenced (in their attitude to
their breasts) by the media, by society. But that's how
society is now. That's life. I'm very doubtful about augment-
ing breasts if it is women's male partners that want them. It
has to be for the women themselves.

The mutterings in the press began in 1991. It worried

some women who came to ask me, 'Am I at risk?' I said to them that this is an American story in origin. So far in the UK we have no evidence of a connection between connective tissue disorders and implants. They haven't proved it in the US. There may be a tiny number of people with a problem where the silicone has leaked. But there are enormous numbers of patients with no problem at all. I may have to revise my advice, but I don't think it's likely.

The image of the plastic surgeon is a problem. But we're not just cosmetic surgeons. Our work is largely reconstructive. One or two people have asked me (after stories of the risks of implants appeared in the press) if I will still be doing breast implants? I have had to justify myself. But I will carry on doing implants. There is not enough evidence for me to stop.

The press coverage has meant an increase in the numbers of anxious women. There was a programme on TV which I didn't see. But from what I heard, it appeared to be rather biased. Most of my sensible patients thought so too.

One does get annoyed as it causes women to be more anxious. You wish people would get their facts straight. It is a shame to put people through so much worry when it is not certain. Breasts are a very sensitive, very important part of women. Last week I took some implants out. The patient was so anxious that she couldn't handle it.

In the eye of the beholder

Cosmetic breast surgery as we know it is a thoroughly modern phenomenon, but across the world, throughout history, people have done bizarre and often damaging things to breasts – often in the name of beauty.

In Spain in the sixteenth and seventeenth centuries, where extreme thinness was fashionable, girls endured lead plates strapped to their chests, so that their breasts would be flattened during puberty.

Amazon women had their right breasts destroyed, making it easier for them to draw a bow and to hunt properly. This was done by making a disc of metal red hot and pressing it on to the right side of the chest during childhood. This damaged the tissue so severely that the breast would never grow.

Some African tribes have traditionally scarred the breasts to 'decorate' them, or have tied them down to make them flat and pendulous. Others have rubbed ointment into the breasts of little girls, fiercely kneading and stretching the nipples to elongate them before binding them with strips of fibre. New Guinean tribes have used nettles and ants to sting the breasts of growing girls to make them swell.

This century, Western women have bound their breasts flat, have thrust them forward and upwards with wired and boned bras, have had their nipples pierced and have submitted to surgery to lift and change their breast shape. Above all, breast implants have become one of the most popular cosmetic operations of modern times. Since 1960, more than two million American women and some 100,000 British women have had implants, around half of them for cosmetic reasons (as opposed to reconstruction after mastectomy). Today, there are still unanswered questions about the safety of such surgery.

Pursuing the illusion

'Beauty', to this generation of women, seems to matter less than it did to our grandmothers, who were more dependent on men and male approval. Yet 'failure' to conform to standards of prettiness – such as having 'normal' breasts – is still a source of great pain to many women, as Jenny and Lesley have testified. You only have to turn on your television to see immediately that women are still valued according to 'beauty': how many female newsreaders are as old and grey as their male colleagues?

But how did we come to our image of beauty? As we have seen, it is not universal: other cultures have preferred breasts to be flat and pendulous, or long and drooping. Naomi Wolf, in her book *The Beauty Myth*, argues that the development of photography had much to do with it. In the 1830s, the new technologies of daguerreotype, tintype and rotogravure were coming into play. The first nude photographs of prostitutes were taken in the 1840s. Advertisements using images of 'beautiful' women first appeared early in Queen Victoria's reign.

Then, as now, 'beautiful' breasts were seen in pictures rather than in the flesh. In the 1990s, breasts of real, ordinary women are still kept covered while bared breasts are mostly confined to porn or pin-ups. These are never long and drooping, never ageing, never the breasts of a lactating mother. We do see real breasts on the TV news, but these are usually the breasts of famine victims from far-away countries, where women are not white and not 'like us'.

Many of today's bared breasts are unreal in another sense too: they may have been trimmed by the scissors of magazine picture editors or artificially changed with the use of 'computer imaging', the technology that can change photographs to make women's bodies appear longer or slimmer.

Breast health articles too are invariably illustrated with glamorous, young breasts. Yet, as Professor Barry Gusterson, director designate of the breast cancer charity, Breakthrough, points out, it is the older breast which is at risk of cancer.

Fashion victims?

Even within the last century, the measurements and characteristics of 'beauty' have shifted many times, and the ideal breast has changed too. In the Roaring Twenties, flappers strapped their breasts down to nothingness. In the 1930s, small, firm breasts à la Jean Harlow were in vogue. By the 1950s the big, cleavaged breasts of Marilyn Monroe had taken over. Breasts were encased in twin cones over a wasp waist and curving hips. By the 1970s the pendulum had swung back again and 'flat-chested', Twiggy-like models were all the rage.

There is an argument that fashion emphasizes breasts at times when women are under pressure to return to traditional 'feminine' roles, as in the 1950s. In her book *Backlash: the Undeclared War Against Women*, American journalist Susan Faludi writes that 'in every backlash [against feminism], the fashion industry has produced punitively restrictive clothing and the fashion press has demanded that women wear it.' She cites a survey in the US which found that clothes which called attention to sexuality – men's or women's – lowered a person's status at the office. Dressing to succeed in business and dressing to be sexually attractive were almost mutually exclusive.

If Faludi is right, today's fashion indicates that we have been in a backlash for some time. During the 1980s breasts were growing steadily more apparent, and by the 1990s the fashion pages were saying – again and again – that breasts were making a comeback. According to journalist Brenda Polan writing in *The Times* (24.10.92):

> The fashion world's latest obsession with breasts has been building for some years. It started back in the early eighties, when Vivienne Westwood put large circular stitched bras over blouses, in tribute to Latin American Indian women, and Jean-Paul Gaultier knitted breasts (complete with crocheted nipples) on to an otherwise simple cable-patterned dress, and then experimented with psychedelic-hued velvet ice-cream cornets set at various unnatural angles.
>
> For several seasons breast-fetishism has been expressed largely through exposed corsetry (the masters being the Italians, Dolce & Gabbana, and Gianni Versace). But while fashion writers could dismiss the catwalk version as unlikely to suit many lifestyles, they could not ignore the influence of a pop icon called Madonna. As a result of Gaultier's labours on her behalf, Madonna turned the well-constructed bra and sturdy corset with suspenders into a statement of a sleazy sort of female power.

Of course Madonna is no fashion victim. If anything, she turns the usual values on their head, and uses her breasts, uses underwear as outerwear, to show that she is strong enough to defy and redefine the rules. Her style and her appeal lie in asserting female power without fear of 'backlash'.

In her wake – but not always carrying her message – came a massive revival for the Gossard Wonderbra, worn by the most fashion-conscious as outerwear. This bra, first introduced in 1968, consists of two lacy, underwired half-cups with little pockets to insert extra padding. A generation which had once thrown their Wonderbras into the flames (apparently, they smouldered horribly), were now witnessing the return of a phenomenon.

At the end of 1991, *Vogue* reported a run on Wonderbras at Fenwick's. Within weeks, the lingerie department was selling a thousand Wonderbras a week. Suddenly, women who never thought they had one were sporting a cleavage. Gossard, who in the 1980s were having to lay people off, began the 1990s able to keep their workforce busy seven days a week. Production of Wonderbras was increased from 4,800 a week to 12,000 a week, and the media dubbed them 'the poor woman's implant'.

Gossard swiftly followed up their success with the 'New Wonderbra'. The *Sun* rejoiced (9.9.92):

> Who needs an expensive boob job when the latest underwear will give you the breast possible shape? First there was the uplift bra. Then came the Gossard Wonderbra. Now get ready for a real storm in a B-cup – the NEW Wonderbra. [This is] the ultimate push-up bra in a three-quarter shape with wide-set shoulder straps, underwiring and light padding to give you extra curves. [The *Sun's* model] is sporting a cleavage like the Grand Canyon.

Breast bonanza

Magazines, newspapers and colour supplements of every variety joined in the breast bonanza with headlines like UP FOR THE CUP, SEDUCTIVE SUPPORT FOR THE BIG GIRLS, PROOF IS IN THE PADDING and BIG, BIGGER, BIGGEST. Of course, each article was lavishly illustrated with 'perfect' breasts.

PARIS OR BUST, read the cover of *Harpers & Queen* (May 1992), across the picture of pouting actress Emmanuelle Beart, her breasts pushed up into an extravagant shelf of flesh. The inside story describes how men mutter, '*Quel balcon*', at the sight.

Not just Europe, but America has been part of the latest breast blitz. The cover of *Newsweek* (25.12.89) showed Dianne Brill (40–23–40) with the new 'Brill' fashion mannequin modelled on her 'ample' dimensions. *Newsweek* announced:

> THE BIGGER THE BETTER: In the '60s it was Twiggy. In the '80s it was Joan Collins. In the '90s it's ... Dianne Brill? That's right, New York night-life's duchess of downtown, the curvaceous actress, model and fashion designer is now 'The Shape of the '90s'. She's been immortalized as a mannequin by Adel Rootstein, who also had produced the Twiggy and Collins models. The choice of Brill proves the bust is back, and the bigger the better. 'It's a Barbie doll fantasy come true,' says Brill. 'I celebrate the ample.'

I must, I must ...

But women's bodies don't spontaneously change at the whim of fashion. You can't take off – or put on – your shape as if it were a miniskirt. So what are the effects on ordinary women of all this breast hype? We are widely judged – and it is hard not to judge ourselves – against these 'perfect' images. We are better liked, considered more attractive, we are even more 'successful' if we are 'good-looking'.

Some of us manage to have confidence in ourselves just as we are, and to let the images wash over us. But not surprisingly, some of us do feel pressure to 'improve' our breasts, turning to 'breast beauty products' with names like Intensive Bust Treatment Programme, Bust Firming Gel or Bust Firming Cream. Not only are these expensive (in the £5–£15 range), but they don't change breast shape.

Yet where there is hope, there are sales. In a survey of young girls for their book *The Breast*, Drs Andrew and Penny Stanway found that 20 per cent of girls had tried to alter their breasts using products like these, as well as exercise (which can slightly lift the breasts through developing the muscle behind them).

Some women take things even further, following the stars of stage and screen onto the operating table. Many models and supermodels have also had breast implants, because they say their livelihoods depend upon it.

But most women who have surgery are not stars or models, just ordinary women – like Lesley and Jenny – who feel a deep sense of dissatisfaction with their bodies. (Naomi Wolf claims one in three women – as compared to one in ten men – falls into this category.) Having surgery is usually more than a matter of superficial 'vanity'. Women have to be prepared to put up with quite a lot of pain to undergo these operations. They usually have to convince surgeons that the operation is for themselves, not to 'please a man'. They may also have to come up with several thousand pounds as it can be difficult to have the operation on the NHS. All this – and in the knowledge that their operations may not even be safe.

Implants: the controversy

For fifty years surgeons have been operating to make women's breasts bigger. They began with pieces of fat taken from the buttocks and inserted into the breasts, but the implanted breasts later shrank or became hard. Next, doctors tried using foam sponges – with a similar lack of success – and then rubber balloons filled with water or saline. But the balloons had a tendency to burst, deflating the breasts.

In the early sixties a sac of gel was pioneered, but the gel sometimes leaked causing painful inflammation of the surrounding tissue. For twenty years, various adaptations of this implant were used, but the problem of breasts hardening around implants remained. Then in the eighties, the polyurethane-coated implant came onto the market, with a much-reduced incidence of hardening. By the beginning of the 1990s, some 5,000 British women were having implants every year, and some two million American women already had implants in place.

Then, in January 1992, the US government agency the Food and Drug Administration (FDA) issued a health warning about implants after hearing that they may be implicated in auto-immune diseases. The FDA called for a halt in the use of silicone breast implants until a panel of experts had examined new evidence on their health risks. The US company that makes most implants and exports them to Britain halted distribution. The company had already been forced to pay $7.34 million (£4m) in damages to a Californian woman who had suffered breast implant rupture. The FDA were also accused of failing to make public the findings of a 1988 study that silicone gel implants caused cancer in 23 per cent of rats.

In Britain, a *World in Action* programme (September 1991) had claimed that two types of implants (MEM and Replicon) were still being used in this country, six months after the Department of Health had advised surgeons not to use them. According to *World in Action*, the polyurethane coating on these implants can bond with body tissues – ultimately causing cancer. *World in Action* also claimed that women weren't being told that 'all implants will leak or bleed very small amounts of silicone continuously while inside the body'.

Plastic surgeons in this country accused the FDA of overreacting and said there was no scientific evidence for the alleged health risks. Women, they complained, had been unnecessarily frightened by alarmist media reports. Breast Cancer Care confirmed that some women with implants in place after mastectomy had been worried and frightened by the reports.

Implants: the risks

Critics of breast implant surgery say the risks include infection, haemorrhage, allergic reaction to anaesthesia, breast hardening, nipple displacement, deflation, rupture and slipping of the implants towards the armpit. Larger breasts can be less sensitive after surgery too, because nerve endings are spaced further apart. Nipples may also be numb.

Implants can mean an end to breastfeeding if milk-producing ducts have been cut. Even when breastfeeding is possible, there may be a chance of leaking silicone entering the breast milk. Feminists have noted that the implant industry is largely carried out by men on women. They ask, 'Why do so few men undergo surgery to "improve" their bodies, while one in fifty American women take the risks of cosmetic breast surgery?'

In her book, *Backlash: the Undeclared War Against Women*, the American journalist Susan Faludi reports that a 1988 US Congressional inquiry revealed major injuries and even deaths from botched implant operations sometimes performed by unqualified 'doctors'. Other US studies found that 15 per cent of cosmetic surgery caused bad scarring, haemorrhaging, nerve damage or other complications. A quarter of all cosmetic surgery in the US was to correct 'errors' in previous surgery. 'For breast implants,' writes Faludi, 'in at least 28 per cent of the cases, repeat surgery was required to remedy the ensuing pain, infection, blood clots or implant ruptures.'

Faludi lists the following as the risks of implant surgery as performed in America:

- Contracture of scar tissue around the implant, separation from the breast tissue and painful hardening of the breast in one-third of cases. Some degree of contracture in 75 per cent of cases.
- Scarring, infection, skin necrosis, blood clots.
- If the implant ruptures, the risks include toxicity, lupus, rheumatoid arthritis and auto-immune diseases like sclerodoma.
- Possible interference with breastfeeding.
- Prevention of detection of breast cancer by concealing breast changes.
- Numbness and loss of sensitivity in the breasts.
- Anaesthesia during surgery has, in one case, resulted in death.

Pounds of flesh

In America, the cosmetic surgery industry is worth a great deal of money. Susan Faludi has described how in the 1960s and 1970s, the ranks of American plastic surgeons quintupled. By 1981, cosmetic surgery was the fastest-growing specialism in American medicine. The surgeons needed more bodies to work on and so they began advertising, seeking publicity for their operations and even offering special credit terms as well as evening and Saturday surgery.

American TV and radio stations gave away free implants. US women's magazines declared that augmentation had become the most popular and widespread operation in America and Europe. Through surgery, they argued, women could 'reinvent' themselves and 'take control' of their lives.

In 1983, reports Faludi, the American Society of Plastic and Reconstructive Surgeons launched a 'practice enhancement' campaign. 'Body sculpturing' was billed as 'safe, effective, affordable and essential to mental health'. The Society also claimed that a body of medical information proved that the 'deformity' of small breasts caused a 'total lack of well-being'.

The campaign worked. By 1988, the case load of qualified cosmetic surgeons in the US had doubled to 750,000 a year. The total number of operations was probably twice that figure. One in sixty American women was spending about $4,000 for breast implants, and by 1987 the average American plastic surgeon was making a profit of $180,000 a year. Nor was all this money coming from rich women: half of the implant patients were women on low incomes who had taken out loans or mortgaged their homes to pay for their operations.

British breasts under the knife

So are we in Britain going to mimic the Americans, climbing on to the operating table by the million? We have followed that culture in so many other ways; we are almost as body-conscious and almost as youth-obsessed. And our attitudes towards sexuality, towards male–female relationships – and towards breasts – are not too different.

In this country, John Terry, managing director of the National Hospital for Aesthetic Plastic Surgery, a private clinic in Bromsgrove, has told the *Independent*: 'Women recognize the value of boobs because they know men are interested in them.'

By 1991, the growing British breast enlargement industry was already worth £20 million a year.

The US embargo on implants seemed to be a setback, but in practice, nothing seemed to change on this side of the Atlantic. Surgeons have continued performing breast augmentations as before, and silicone implants have never been banned in this country.

The British Association of Aesthetic Plastic Surgeons (BAAPS) stands by this statement:

> BAAPS is confident of the safety of silicone implants and wishes to reassure any patient with these devices that they have no cause for concern. Unless a woman is having problems with her implants we are not recommending that she have them removed. If she is having symptoms and feels they may be related to her implant, she should contact the surgeon who carried out her operation.

BAAPS, which has 140 member surgeons, is at the reputable end of the plastic surgery spectrum. Its procedures (BAAPS members have to be contacted through GPs and so have access to women's medical records) are designed to make sure that women who need it get referred for psychiatric care. 'Dysmorphia', explains a BAAPS spokesperson, 'is a form of mental illness in which women repeatedly turn to surgery to alleviate their physical self-hatred.'

But not all surgeons act in women's best interests when large amounts of money are involved. Many of the private clinics – of the kind which regularly advertise in women's magazines – use surgeons who are not members of BAAPS. They have been accused of using hard-sell tactics on women who would be better off getting psychiatric treatment. There are stories of women who take a friend for support in inquiring about breast surgery – and *both* women come out of the clinic with implanted breasts.

Beyond beauty

Yet we have never been quite as knife-happy, nor quite as obsessed with perfection, as the Americans. Many of the women I spoke to for this book are independent-minded and individual in their attitudes to fashion: they feel free to pick and choose from the latest styles, camping it up in a Wonderbra for a party perhaps, but dressing from Oxfam at other times.

And many British women (and men) still have a commonsense dislike of the idea of cosmetic breast surgery. Judy Skinner, writing in Somerset's *Justwomen* magazine, describes how she was shocked by the attitude of a male visitor from Florida who told her:

You can tell the girls who've had them because when they lie down by the pool their breasts still keep pointing upwards. Otherwise it's quite difficult. I've been out with loads of girls who've had them and I often didn't know until they told me.

While not dismissing the genuine feelings of many women who say cosmetic breast surgery has changed their lives, we can still hope for a different sort of change. Surgeons have argued that it is quicker and easier to change a woman's breasts than it is to change society. But changing society would mean less pain and risk for women – although more for some cosmetic surgeons, financially speaking.

We can start by personally rejecting attitudes that say only young and pert is beautiful. We can challenge the prevalence of pin-ups and page-three pictures which promote these attitudes. We can – through books like this one – discover some truths about breasts, pass them on to our daughters, discuss them with our friends and menfolk, and accept our own breasts as uniquely ours. And when we get the chance we can show that breasts have more than just the one, sexual, role. Narrow, fashion-dictated standards of 'beauty' undervalue women.

Our breasts have another sort of beauty: the natural, active, priceless beauty of being able to sustain human life.

4
The battle for breastfeeding

If the breast is a battleground, the greatest battles rage across it when women give birth. We live in a bottle-feeding society, and a woman's choice to use her breasts for feeding can trigger enormous conflicts.

Suddenly the breast as sex symbol is challenged by the breast as baby-feeder. Suddenly the idea that it is sexy to show a bit of breast is turned upside down, and showing a bit of breast can mean humiliating exile from public places.

New fathers, new grannies, health professionals and formula manufacturers all join the fray, making judgements, passing comment and pulling the emotions of the new mother every which way. The new mother, who may never have seen anyone else breastfeed, tries valiantly to learn this skill, but she is badly advised and hampered by those who should help her.

It is sad, but not surprising, that most women in this country give up within weeks, leaving us with one of the lowest breast-feeding rates in Europe. Many determined women do carry on, however, with inestimable benefits to their babies and themselves.

This chapter looks at the experience of breastfeeding from a woman's point of view, describing the conflicts, the complications – and the joys – of breastfeeding today.

Ideal milk

It is a kind of miracle: a woman brings new life into the world, and immediately she has the power to nourish, comfort and satisfy her baby with her breasts.

The myths of many civilizations have celebrated the life-giving powers of the breast. The Greeks believed the stars of the Milky Way were formed from drops of Juno's breast milk. Artemis of Ephesus – who had many breasts – was the universal wetnurse, the source of abundance and fertility for all life on earth. The Egyptian goddess Hathor, creator of the universe, was depicted as a cow. So great were the properties of her milk that kings would suckle at her breasts.

It is an ancient belief that milk production is connected to spiritual or supernatural forces, and nursing mothers in many parts of the world have worn amulets to boost their milk supply. In Christianity, the milk of Mary, mother of Jesus, has carried many complex spiritual meanings. Mary's milk has been seen as an emanation from Heaven, a symbol of sustenance for the soul; it has meant wisdom, love, mercy and healing.

The emotional and spiritual power of breastfeeding is the theme of an old story which crops up in many cultures, across many centuries. For instance, in Roman legend, Micon was saved from death by starvation in prison because his daughter Pero visited him every day and kept him alive with her breast milk. In John Steinbeck's *The Grapes of Wrath*, Rose of Sharon saves a starving man's life in the moving last scene of the novel as she lies down beside him to feed him with her breast milk.

And as far back as Homer, stories have been told in which breast milk symbolizes life. In the *Iliad*, Hecuba, mother of Hector, bares her breast to her son to remind him of how he once suckled there as she begs him not to go into battle against Achilles.

Many societies have also believed that breast milk has magical healing qualities, and breast milk has been used as a medicine for all sorts of ailments, ranging from deafness to snakebite. In Nepal, women massage their babies with breast milk to promote their health and well-being. British mothers have told me they use drops of breast milk to cure 'sticky eye' in their babies (breast milk does, in fact, have powerful anti-viral properties). Sheila Kitzinger, the internationally renowned expert on breast-feeding and childbirth, adds that Caribbean women use breast milk to cure eye injuries and infections.

Unique properties

This century science has come up with proof of what people have always known: that breast milk has uniquely valuable properties. Nutritionally, there is nothing to match it. Breastfed babies need no other food or drink for the first four to six months of life. Breast milk also protects babies against many diseases such as asthma, eczema, gastro-enteritis, diabetes, pneumonia, ear infections, polio and other conditions.

Even in the UK, where formula milk can be made up with clean water (in contrast to many countries), a bottle-fed baby is up to ten times more likely to suffer from gastro-intestinal illnesses than a breastfed one. Breastfed babies are also less likely to be victims of cot death. The latest research also suggests that breast milk is good for a baby's brain, containing elements which are essential for brain growth, especially in premature babies.

Breastfeeding is good for women's health too. Not only does it help women to get their figures back more quickly after childbirth, but women who breastfeed may have a lower risk of ovarian and breast cancer.

Apart from the proven physical advantages, there are also immeasurable emotional benefits which flow from breastfeeding, for both mother and child. The baby lies warm against the mother's skin, absorbing love along with the nourishment, hearing her heart beat, making a relationship to last a lifetime. The mother, too, grows in pride and self-confidence while watching her baby develop. This is how breastfeeding women describe the experience:

> You feel so close, linked in a special way which allows you to provide for all their needs.

> For four months he had nothing but breast milk and I felt the baby was 'all my own work'.

> Breastfeeding gives you time to just sit and be with the baby. It's also convenient – at night you can lie down with the baby and drift off to sleep – and it's free.

> It means that birth is not the sudden end of the child-bearing process. Breastfeeding becomes a gentle way of weaning yourself off the baby.

> You're so needed. You become a life-support machine.

> Babies take the breast so happily, accepting and loving everything, accepting and loving you.

> Babies are more secure when you breastfeed them. If they can depend on you when they're young, they can be independent later.

> It's so wonderful, it's indescribable.

In the real world

Ideally then breastfeeding is a profoundly loving, health-giving and fulfilling experience for mother and baby alike. Yet, in reality, this is not always the case.

For three generations in the West, bottle-feeding has been taking over from breastfeeding. According to Chloe Fisher, a clinical specialist who now runs a clinic for baby-feeding problems at the John Radcliffe Hospital in Oxford:

> The history of what has happened to breastfeeding is mind-blowing. Men invented rules for breastfeeding, with no clue of how the process works. The art of breastfeeding has been all but lost. Most of the information women are now given is complete poppycock, based on the teaching at the turn of the century which supposed the breast was a bottle. Health professionals don't realize how desperately the women in their care need information and support.
>
> The most common problem is that women don't understand how the baby draws the breast into its mouth. Women are given advice such as 'put the nipple into the baby's mouth' – as if the breast were a bottle – but that's disastrous, because it stops the baby lapping in the breast tissue. Breastfeeding today is a right old mess. We now have good information, but there is a lack of will to use it (on the part of health professionals), because it means admitting you were wrong previously.

Not a piece of cake

At a social level, too, there are big problems for women who want to breastfeed (and most mothers do want to satisfy this powerful, physiological need, believes Chloe Fisher). We live surrounded by images of breasts which most of us find embarrassing and degrading. We grow up with the idea that breasts are for sex. Not surprisingly, women can find it very difficult to shake off the image of breasts as objects of lust and laughter in order to use them for feeding:

> There's something sick about a society that daily shows women's breasts in its newspapers – but doesn't let us breastfeed.

Often women themselves are opposed to breastfeeding. They fear, with good grounds, that 'people won't like it'. They are confused by the taboos about breastfeeding and disturbed by its 'animal' nature:

> There is something bovine about it, like being part of a milking parlour.

> My daughter-in-law didn't want to breastfeed because she said it made her feel like a dog or a cat.

Besides which, we have learned that breasts are 'sexual' and we mustn't be 'sexual' with our babies. For some women, breastfeeding is an intensely pleasurable experience and yet, deep down, we have absorbed the notion that such pleasure is 'bad'. Certainly many men find the idea that the baby's sucking gives 'their' woman pleasure very disturbing.

We are confused about what is 'sexual' and what is 'sensual'. This confusion is heightened by today's crisis over child sexual abuse. And in addition to the sex taboos, food is a very emotive subject for women in our diet-obsessed society. In breastfeeding, food and sex overlap: it may all be too much for some women, and most give up within weeks of starting to breastfeed.

The down side: soreness, tiredness and depression

On the practical level, too, breastfeeding is not easy for women. Mary Renfrew, director of the Midwifery Research Programme at the National Perinatal Epidemiology Unit (and herself a mother), puts it like this:

> Women often do run into real difficulties with breastfeeding, and there is often no place to turn for help. Physically, it is a very hard thing to do, and it is a difficult skill to learn. There may also be anxiety about the baby; when it cries you wonder if you are doing the right things. Women suffer from a lack of confidence that it is possible to sustain life this way. Breastfed babies also wake up more at night, and they feed more often than bottle-fed babies. Mothers who breastfeed do get less sleep than other mothers, and they do get more depressed.

When women don't have the opportunity to learn the skills of breastfeeding from each other – and few do – things can go disastrously wrong, especially when they have received misguided advice:

> I experienced incredible soreness with scabs on my nipples. It hurt more than the birth. It was toe-curlingly awful. I had to have a

paracetamol and a glug of sherry before I started. I was on the verge of giving up until a breastfeeding counsellor helped me to carry on. And I was determined to do it: I'm not ever giving up now!

It hurt. For four months it was painful. My toes curled. And I had the feeling that I was being drained, sucked dry. With my second baby I stopped after a week and that was it.

Even those of us who do manage to get into the swing of breastfeeding and to keep it up for four or six or nine months do sometimes admit relief when the whole thing is over:

As much as I loved breastfeeding, I must admit I was very glad when I could wear my shirt down for the entire day. I got really fed up with all that unbuttoning and buttoning up again ... I just wanted my body back.

Women who don't breastfeed, usually because they have met too many difficulties, may be doubly penalized: they feel not only 'failure', but guilt because of that 'failure'.

I felt worse when breastfeeding was the 'right on' thing to do. You feel such a failure if you actually can't breastfeed very effectively. I felt more at other people's mercy than when I stopped.

Sadly, many women stop breastfeeding long before they would really like to because of pain and the fear of insufficient milk. Yet with the right help (see Chapter Five) there is no reason why they shouldn't carry on as long as they want to.

Sexy or saggy?

The 'topless' and pornographic images of breasts that surround us add to the confusion. When the MP Clare Short launched her bill to ban topless pictures in tabloid newspapers she received letters like this one, concerned at how porn has made women deeply uncomfortable with their own breasts, and therefore less inclined to breastfeed:

> I think the effects of pornography are more widespread than first appears. As a health visitor, I encourage breastfeeding, but am aware of the unnatural and unhealthy attitude women have towards their own breasts. They are almost taboo for their owners. It's as if they are not a part of the woman's self. They are the property of the man in the relationship. I feel this is in part responsible for the low take-up of breastfeeding in less-educated women.

The artificial standard of 'perfection' set up by topless pictures also makes women ashamed of their own real breasts. As this midwife said:

> Some women don't want to expose their breasts because they feel they are too big – or too small. Quite often when you talk to these women you find it is their husbands who have influenced them, and that they have come to see their breasts as a sexual organ belonging to their man, not to their baby.

In a world where women's popularity, relationships – even their financial security – may rest upon living up to a standard of 'perfection', they fear 'losing their figures'. There is a widespread belief that in feeding a baby, a woman's breasts will grow 'ugly'. Marlene Dietrich is reputed to have accused her daughter

Maria of ruining her breasts, calling her a greedy child who sucked too much.

In 1992, the *Sun* ran a feature about the television presenter Amanda de Cadanet which exploited this fear and reinforced the idea that the only good breasts are pre-fertile breasts. Under the headline HOW AMANDA DE SAGANET [sic] CAN RESCUE HER BOOBS it launched this attack:

> It's motherhood or bust! New mum Amanda de Cadanet has found out she can't have both. Her once pert 34B boobs are sagging since she gave birth to Atlanta four months ago. We reckon the 20-year-old blonde is now a 38D.

A 'before' picture showed Amanda in a corset top – 'before her baby ... *so sexy*' – compared to an 'after' picture of Amanda squashed into a boob tube: 'four months after the birth, her boobs drooping ... *so saggy*'. They followed up with detailed instructions on how Amanda (and all women) can improve their bustline with exercises.

In fact, the changes in breasts that come with motherhood are caused by pregnancy, not by breastfeeding. And breastfeeding, which causes the uterus to shrink, actively helps a woman to regain her pre-birth waistline.

Besides, why are we so squeamish about the fact that our breasts change with motherhood? They have changed with puberty. They will change after menopause. It is entirely natural – or is that what worries us?

'Saggy' is only an insult in a society such as ours where the only 'beautiful' woman has the body of a teenager. In some cultures, the opposite is true. There is a witches' curse from Papua New Guinea which condemns the victim's breasts to 'stay pert and upright like a young girl's for ever'. And Sheila Kitzinger tells me that in some cultures women wish for long breasts – so that they can toss them over a shoulder to feed an infant while they work. Admittedly, we don't need this skill as we sit at our office desks, but our idea of the beautiful breast is by no means universal.

Unfortunately we have exported many of our attitudes to other countries, with lethal consequences for many babies. Chloe Fisher reported from a tour of war-torn Croatia that breastfeeding had been replaced by bottle-feeding on 'aesthetic' (i.e. 'beauty') grounds.

Curfew on mothers

Our culture's defection to bottle-feeding dates back to the turn of the century, when three out of four women of the upper social classes were turning to bottles. It was amongst the 'lower orders' that the animal-like function of breastfeeding survived. There was a widespread belief that increasing civilization would mean an end to breastfeeding. And as working-class women realized that bottle-feeding was preferred by their 'betters', they followed suit.

By the late 1960s, breastfeeding was almost destroyed in the USA and was at a low ebb in this country. It was middle-class, educated women who – backed by scientific evidence – decided they wanted to breastfeed again, but they remain a minority. Within half a century there had been a complete turnaround in the social class of breastfeeding women.

There are still tremendous pressures not to breastfeed in public. It seems ridiculous to us that Victorian women were obliged to hide their pregnant bodies from public view. But today's breastfeeding mothers have to struggle against an equivalent curfew when their babies are small:

> I don't go out for long because I don't feel I can breastfeed in public, so I spend hours and hours alone with my newborn baby. As a mother, you become an outsider.

At a time when women are already at risk from depression, breastfeeding mothers are made to feel as if they can't go out. Or if they do go out – and breastfeed – they can be made to feel like pariahs. As this woman wrote to Clare Short:

> When I breastfeed my four-month-old son, I ensure that it is done as discreetly as possible. I do not 'bare all' to the world. Yet in one large department store, my friend and I were asked to stop as it 'wasn't very nice for the other customers'. In all fairness the staff did provide us with a room where we could eat and feed our babies, but it didn't stop us feeling like social outcasts.

Not surprisingly the phrase that comes up most when talking to breastfeeding women is 'I was determined' – and many do carry on successfully in defiance of the obstacles:

> Travelling by train or plane with babies is tricky if you're shy of breastfeeding in front of other people. But I have my own strategy now: when he gets hungry we go into the first-class seats which are quieter and more roomy. I have never been challenged: perhaps people are too embarrassed!

> When I first had to feed my baby on a London bus, I avoided people's eyes and looked out of the window. But now I'm very blasée about it. It's astonishing how few people even notice. It's no great performance.

A dirty business?

Picture an adult customer of a restaurant being packed off to feed in the toilet. It would be insulting, unhygienic, inconceivable. Yet it happens to babies all the time. According to a 1989 National Childbirth Trust survey of restaurants that claimed they provided facilities for breastfeeding mothers, 70 per cent provided no more than a toilet:

> I was having dinner with some friends in a London bistro. My baby was about two months old and when she became fractious I began to feed her, aware of the fact that the low light and the high pews we sat on would make it difficult for anyone else to see. But within minutes the manager was at our table. Other diners had complained, he said. If I had to feed the baby, I could go upstairs to the toilet. After an embarrassing argument, I went up to the toilet because the baby was crying. I'll never forget the humiliation of sitting in that white cubicle with my baby as if we were doing something dirty. Immediately afterwards we all left the restaurant.

When a woman breastfeeds her baby she is behaving as if she has the right to use her own body as she chooses, as if it is her choice when and how she exposes her breasts. This can make people very upset. It is all very well for the male-controlled porn industry or the tabloid press to expose women's breasts for sexual purposes, but woe betide the woman who exposes her own in public for baby-feeding purposes.

Sheila Kitzinger believes that sending breastfeeding women off to toilets is more than a mere matter of convenience or embarrassment on the part of restaurant managers. It has deeper cultural echoes of ancient 'pollution' beliefs about women's bodily fluids. Kitzinger says:

> Breast milk has long been associated with excretion. It is thought of as an unclean fluid. There is also a fear of the power of breast milk. It has the power to sustain life – and men fear it in the same way that they may fear menstrual blood.

The breast, believes Kitzinger, is seen as a dangerous place because it is a powerful place. Kitzinger argues that, like the vagina, the breast is one of women's feared and secret bodily 'weapons' which threaten the male identity.

Doctors (mostly men) have extended the idea of the 'threat' to include babies. In her book *The Politics of Breastfeeding*, Gabrielle Palmer describes how doctors have traditionally treated breast-feeding as a potentially suffocating process (the suffocating breast is a recurrent male fantasy – see Chapter Two):

> A widespread recommendation which persists to this day is to hold the nipple and breast between the fingers in case the baby cannot breathe. [Yet] there is not a single case of a baby being suffocated by the breast. In fact a baby *has* to be close to the breast in order to feed well, and human noses – with nostrils to the side – are perfectly constructed for breathing while breast-feeding.

The notion of breast milk being dangerous because it is contaminated is as ancient as it is international. In AD 200, the physician Soranus advised women not to breastfeed their babies for three weeks after birth as the recently delivered woman is 'ill', and her milk is 'thick, indigestible and raw'. And in Zulu tradition a man risked losing his virility if a drop of breast milk should fall on his skin.

In hospitals across Europe, women may still be separated from their babies for 'hygiene' reasons, the assumption being that the mother (as opposed to midwives, doctors and visitors) is a carrier of germs. And traditionally, women's nipples have been 'washed' before they feed babies (stripping them of their protective secretions in the process).

According to one midwife from Taunton:

> They used to put Gentian violet on nipples here to disinfect them. It has been banned now because of the potentially carcinogenic [cancer causing] effect.

And according to this mother of three:

> They taught us that when you finish feeding you must always carefully wipe off your nipples to stop them getting sore. In fact the reverse is true.

In Moscow, says Sheila Kitzinger, the nipples of breastfeeding women are routinely painted with disinfectant iodine.

The pollution myth is also the basis for apocryphal tales like this one: Nurses on a maternity unit offer a young doctor a cup of coffee. He gratefully accepts and drinks it down. Then they tell him they had whitened it with breast milk, expressed by women on the ward. Exit doctor, in state of shock.

Someone else's breast milk?

Yet we are all affected at some level by the breast milk taboo – or why else do so many of us blanch at the idea of our babies being fed by another woman. Perhaps there are other factors at work too – like the current fear of AIDS, like the modern sense that children are exclusively their parents' property. But it is remarkable that, until this century, wet-nursing was widely accepted in this country. Yet few women these days are happy with the idea of another woman feeding their baby:

> A friend once offered to feed my baby if she cried while I was out. I suddenly decided not to go out.

> I don't think I would mind if my sister were to feed my baby. And I wouldn't mind feeding hers if it cried and she wasn't there. But it has never happened, no. And I think we would ask each other's permission first.

> I wouldn't like it unless it was a very close friend or relative.

In a scene in the 1992 television comedy *Absolutely Fabulous* Jennifer Saunders tells her screen daughter that she was breastfed as a baby. The daughter's face shows disbelief, then disgust – then horror – as Saunders admits they lived in a commune at the time, and that breastfeeding was, well, also communal . . .

Contrast many Third World countries, where babies are regularly fed by other women – aunts, grandmothers, cousins – in the mother's absence. A film made by the anthropologist Margaret Mead on a Balinese island shows that in some cultures even fathers will provide a nipple to soothe a crying baby.

During a *Woman's Hour* broadcast on breasts, the story emerged of an African matriarch who was making a speech to her people from a public platform. Just below her a baby was crying noisily, making it difficult for people to hear her speech. The speaker reached into the crowd, grasped the baby and put it to her own breast. Not only did she win instant silence from the child, but she won the wild applause of her audience who took her action to symbolize a leader's relationship with her people.

Yet even a woman as well-informed as Sheila Kitzinger admits to some qualms on the sharing of breast milk. She laughs as she describes how she once went into the kitchen of an Oxford boarding house to find the earth-motherly landlady expressing milk from her breast into the cake-mixture on the table. Kitzinger admits she rather went off the landlady's cakes after that. She said, 'I found them to be rather sweet!'

Not *still* feeding, are you?

There are also rules about how long to breastfeed which differ strongly from one culture to another. In many Third World countries it is normal for women to feed children for three or four years. But in Britain, the norm is far less, although it varies between social groups.

At one end of the scale is the mother (she is in the majority) who tries to feed her baby, but after a few weeks, stops. It is widely accepted that she has 'done her best' and 'had a go', but her milk is 'insufficient' or of 'poor quality'. (These are myths.) Rather than being helped to breastfeed properly, this mother is usually encouraged to turn to the bottle, for the baby's sake.

At the next level is the woman who fully breastfeeds for a few months and then starts the baby on solids while keeping on with night feeds until about six to nine months. She tends to be the middle-class mother who is at home, or doing some part-time work. As long as she stops feeding her baby in public before it is 'too big' (i.e. old enough to wear shoes), she will generally be approved of as a 'good mother'.

Then there are the mothers – mostly found in support groups like the La Lèche League and the Association of Breastfeeding Mothers – who carry on breastfeeding until their children are toddlers or of school age. It is this group which faces the most disapproval:

People are always saying – you're not *still* feeding him are you? They look at me as if I am a pariah. They think it's dirty. Some ask – what does your husband think of it?

People think – especially if your baby is a boy – that there must be something sexual in it.

It's the idea that the child will consciously ask for the breast, walking over and lifting your shirt, that people find distasteful.

My daughter was virtually swinging on the light and I was still feeding her. Somebody actually said to me, 'She doesn't want to feed any more', and she didn't. So we stopped at fifteen months although I could have gone on for ever.

As a midwife, I knew two women who went on breastfeeding for years. Both had been told they would never have children and the babies were incredibly precious to them.

But there are questions asked behind a woman's back if she breastfeeds for 'too long'. Is she doing it to keep power in the family? To exclude her husband? For her own satisfaction? Whatever the answers, many other cultures in the world wouldn't even ask the questions.

The granny factor

These accumulated taboos and inhibitions also contribute to what researchers have dubbed 'the granny factor'. Many new mothers, fresh from hospital, have their mothers, or mothers-in-law, to 'help' them through those exhausting early weeks. Yet today's grannies probably had their own babies during the sixties when bottle-feeding was very much in fashion, and they seem – sometimes unconsciously – hostile to breastfeeding.

Perhaps some grannies are sensitive to the implicit criticism that bottle-feeding ('it was good enough for my children') isn't as good as breastfeeding. The new generation of mothers may seem to be having a dig at the old. Or grannies may want to protect their own daughters from the disappointment they experienced in 'failing' to breastfeed.

In a study from Newcastle Polytechnic (*Independent*, 29.12.92) the question which best determined which women were most likely to give up breastfeeding early was, 'How often do you see your mother?' The *more* often women saw their mothers, the *less* likely they were to breastfeed.

Many women have tales to tell about negative remarks from their own mothers:

> My family were gathered together for a wedding in a big hotel. I was sitting in the corner of a quiet lounge when my baby needed feeding, so I discreetly got started without anyone noticing. My mother, after telling me that I should go upstairs to my room in order to feed, stood up and made a public apology for my shameless behaviour. She succeeded in attracting everyone's attention to what I was doing.

> After a few months of breastfeeding, my mother started to tell me that it was time for me to stop. She argued that the baby was 'draining me dry', 'sapping my strength', and so on.

> My mother says things like – you're one of the lucky ones who can feed. But are you sure it's good enough milk? Are you sure you shouldn't be topping her up with a bottle?

> My mother-in-law is appalled whenever I breastfeed. She says, 'Oh,

not again! Surely she can't be hungry!' The idea that my baby
might want to suck for comfort, or for pleasure, doesn't occur to
her: breast milk should be there purely to nourish the baby!

Yet women of the previous generation were themselves subject
to enormous pressures either not to breastfeed, or to breastfeed
strictly in private. Many say they 'couldn't breastfeed'. Others
say their husbands wanted them not to. Inevitably they have
strong feelings on the subject, varying from disgust to long-
buried disappointment. Inevitably they have passed on an emotional legacy:

> I fed from the breasts of my own mother: I find that an uncomfort-
> able thought.

> Breasts and breastfeeding were never discussed at home. I don't
> know if I was breastfed or not.

> My mother had twelve children and she breastfed all of them.
> However, I never saw her breastfeeding. She used to take the baby
> away into the bedroom to do it. When we were little we thought
> she was killing the baby.

Other family members of the older generation can be just as
negative about breastfeeding:

> My father came to visit me in the hospital when my baby was
> born. But when I started to feed her, he couldn't even look at me.
> He couldn't even talk.

> When I started to feed my baby on a family visit, my mother-in-law
> banished me to another room so that her [unmarried] son wouldn't
> see me doing it.

> I have found it very hard to feed in front of my brother, and in
> front of my father.

The only person I felt uncomfortable in front of was my father. It's because I am still 'his little girl'.

Male claims

Some of the blame for breastfeeding failures also lies at the door of this generation of fathers. There is the kind of man who simply feels that his partner's breasts belong to him and that the baby should not be allowed to get in the way. He can't cope with the dual – sexual and maternal – role of the breast. He is disturbed by the notion that his partner might actually enjoy feeding the baby (the old idea that it is mucky for women to enjoy their bodies still lingers):

He kept saying – surely it's not natural for you to enjoy it, is it?

He would say at about weekly intervals – don't you think it's time you started to wean her now? I sensed that he was very jealous.

As a midwife I have found that the main reason women give up breastfeeding is opposition from their male partners. How women get on does very much depend on the kind of support they get from their men. But a lot of men are jealous. It's like men watching other women on the beach: it's all right as long as their own wife or girlfriend has a bikini top on. They want to look, but they don't want other men to look. It's a possessive thing.

But there is also New Man, who wants to express himself emotionally by feeding the baby – and so he encourages his partner to 'get the baby on to the bottle'. The bottle, however, is not best for the baby's health. And New Man has to be politely reminded that there are other things he can do for the baby (perhaps at baby's other end?). There are many years of involvement with his child yet to come:

> There is another kind of jealousy which men experience when it comes to breastfeeding. As a midwife I did come across one man who was really jealous because he wanted to be able to feed the baby himself. He was trying to stop her from breastfeeding and she did eventually give up because of it.

Men need educating about breastfeeding as much as women do. In Scandinavia men attend breastfeeding classes. It's no coincidence that almost all women there leave hospital breastfeeding and most breastfeed for six months.

Many a man is also unsettled by the deep-seated incest taboo: his lover has become a mother (like his own mother) – and anyway, what is he supposed to feel when milk squirts from his partner's nipples when he sucks them, or when she reaches orgasm? Women can be equally embarrassed by their newly liquid lovemaking. (It happens because the same hormone, oxytocin, which controls the let-down reflex in breastfeeding is also involved in sexual arousal and orgasm.)

And many men, if they are honest, fear that their woman will declare her breasts off-limits to him until the baby has finished with them. How galling, how frustrating to be usurped by a guzzling infant!:

> I wouldn't let my husband go near them for as long as I was breastfeeding. They were definitely the baby's territory. The rest of my body was available to him, but not my breasts.

> I didn't want mine touched for fear they would leak.

No sex please, we're breastfeeding

Some men do discover that their sex life has been put on hold in the breastfeeding months either because their female partners lose the desire for sex – or because *they* do. Michel Odent, author of *The Nature of Birth and Breastfeeding*, makes the general observation (which some people may not agree with) that:

> A woman who is breastfeeding is not receptive to the demands of the male, and the male is not attracted to breastfeeding females. This produces a conflict of interest.

The *Independent* (8.7.92) has explored the frustration, hurt and disappointment that some new fathers feel when the baby arrives – but sex departs. One postnatal counsellor reported that 40 per cent of the first-time mothers she sees have no sexual relations with their husbands for up to two years. While the exhaustion experienced by new mothers is probably the main reason, breastfeeding can also lower the libido in causing the release of the hormone prolactin.

This can put intense strain upon marriages, which are more prone to breaking down in the eighteen months after birth than at any other time. As one father put it:

> It's not just a sexual thing. It's the fact that my wife puts my daughter first, second and third and that I come a poor fourth. The child is satisfying all her needs and her lack of interest in sex has become a metaphor for her disinterest in me.

Some women also say they don't really feel like having sex in the breastfeeding months:

> I still enjoy it, but the hunger has gone.

> You feel different when you are breastfeeding. You are different –

> even your vaginal secretions are different. When you stop breastfeeding it changes; you can stop giving so much to the baby and start giving more to your partner.

Women are certainly under pressure to get back to 'normal' (i.e. 'sexual') as soon as possible after birth. Even the maternity wards have exercise charts to tell women how to 'get their figures back', and within days of the birth doctors and/or midwives will be asking the new mother what she is going to do about contraception.

> There was a point, within a week after he was born, when I thought – if one more midwife or doctor asks me what I am going to do about contraception, I will scream.

But some women – and men – find that breastfeeding has the effect of enhancing sex. Many women say that it is postnatal tiredness, rather than any consequences of breastfeeding, that is the real enemy of sex. Breastfeeding a baby can make a woman feel sexier and help her enjoy her breasts more:

> I have a friend who says that breastfeeding is the most wonderful sexual experience she has ever had – and she says this in front of her own husband too! No wonder she goes into a separate room to feed!

> A baby sucking on your nipples feels rather like anyone else sucking on your nipples. It can be very exciting.

> If you are happy to breastfeed you get a very positive view of your body which helps you sexually.

Men, too, are just as likely to find the bigger breasts of their partner a newly discovered sexual bonus:

Some men want to taste your breast milk.

My husband liked the fact that my breasts were bigger. I rather enjoyed it too . . .

Medical hurdles

The traditions and structure of the health service can work against successful breastfeeding, too. The story of the decline of breastfeeding the world over is a story of a male-dominated medical profession taking over the management of childbirth and infant feeding.

In the West it has had a significant sub-plot: at the turn of the century, the mechanization of the dairy industry led to a large surplus of whey products. In a triumph of marketing over common sense, these surpluses were turned into artificial milk and women were encouraged to pay for what no one had ever paid them to do in the past.

The impact of these historical developments is still very much felt by any woman who gives birth in a British hospital today. All too often, midwives and other health professionals impose unnecessary restrictions on breastfeeding from the very moment of birth:

I wanted to have the baby in bed with me so that I could feed her on the night that she was born. But the midwife got really angry with me, said I would get sore nipples, and eventually stormed off, drawing the curtains angrily round me. I didn't get sore nipples.

I didn't get to cuddle or feed mine for hours after he was born.

Then I got sore nipples, and was never able to enjoy it. I tried to carry on for two months, but the midwives kept saying, 'If it's not working, go on the bottle.' I did eventually, and within days I wished I hadn't. I missed the closeness. I fed my second baby successfully for nine months. [Women who put their babies to the breast within an hour of birth are twice as likely to carry on feeding as those who don't. *Independent*, 29.12.92]

Even in the hospital, as soon as women started feeding, the nurses would ask, 'Do you want the screens?', and hide you away.

The midwives ask you, 'What do you want to do, dear?' As if breastfeeding has no particular advantages over bottle-feeding. I think that's unforgivable.

Some midwives and health visitors, of course, are marvellously supportive, spending as much time as they can in counselling women on how best to breastfeed. Nor are midwives responsible for the chronic underfunding of the NHS which leaves a shortage of their number in most hospital wards.

The training of health professionals also leaves a lot to be desired. Extraordinary though it may seem, many midwives may get no more than a day's training in breastfeeding and GPs may get no more than one hour. Health care for new mothers is also very fragmented, and as one midwife leaves her shift to be replaced by another, no single health worker is taking responsibility for how she gets on:

When I was a young midwife I did everything from the book, I thought it would help mothers. I was much better at helping mothers breastfeed after I'd done it myself. Most midwives are not mothers; a lot of them are in training, and once you get good at the job, up the ladder you go into administration.

> The advice I gave out as a midwife before I had my own children was totally off the wall. I was teaching women to feed for two minutes on each side and no more for the first day, every four hours, and so on. It seems incredible to me now!

Breastfeeding is not an instinct, it is a learned skill, and today's new mother may never have seen anyone else do it. Without proper support, how is she to know how to position the baby properly at the breast to avoid the sore and cracked nipples which can make breastfeeding an agony? How is she to know that the fat-rich milk which provides the calories the baby needs come at the end of a feed and that the baby needs a good mouthful of breast as well as nipple – and unrestricted feeding – in order to get this milk?

The growing trend for shorter and shorter stays in hospital also means that many women leave before the end of the critical first week in which breastfeeding – and the confidence to continue breastfeeding – needs to be established.

And the baby-milk manufacturers are always on the scene, ready to take advantage of women's fears that they don't have enough milk to successfully feed their babies. Although the WHO and UNICEF have an International Code of marketing which bans all forms of promotion of baby milk, baby-milk companies regularly offer big financial carrots to hospitals. According to one newspaper report (*Independent*, 29.12.92), Farley's recently offered UK hospitals £18 for every baby fed on Ostermilk, and a lump sum of £24,000 if all were fed on it and mothers persuaded to continue with it when they left.

Mary Renfrew argues that the advertising of breast milk substitutes has been hugely important in the decline of breastfeeding:

There is a lot of very persuasive, glossy advertising of new baby milks, teats, bottles, follow-on milks and weaning foods. These play on women's most vulnerable emotions and undermine their confidence in continuing to feed. The baby-milk companies are not allowed to give away free samples, but the hospitals buy in the milk which is readily available, sitting on the lockers in sweet little bottles.

But, says Chloe Fisher, midwives and doctors have let baby-milk manufacturers get away with it:

The baby-milk industry has been very powerful, but many members of my profession have also been very gullible. The manufacturers have moved into the space which we've created for them.

The international picture

Internationally – and the West has led the way in this – bottle-feeding has been a major disaster. In parts of the world where the water supply is unsafe for drinking, and where mothers are unable to sterilize feeding equipment, bottle-feeding causes infections like diarrhoea, which is the biggest killer of children worldwide.

An estimated one and a half million babies die every year because they are not breastfed. Millions more become ill as a result of bottle-feeding. James Grant, director of UNICEF, has said that 'the resulting death toll is equivalent to that from the Hiroshima explosion in 1945'. According to UNICEF, babies are up to 25 times more likely to die if they are bottle-fed.

In poor families of the developing world, the expense of formula milk (it often costs more than half the entire family income) means that other children have to go hungry. The temptation for poor mothers is to dilute the formula to make it go further – but this means that not even the baby is being adequately fed. Tragically, in encouraging dependency on a product that brings hunger, the West has persuaded women to renounce their own invaluable natural resource: mothers who are themselves starving can still produce enough milk for their babies.

The baby-milk companies stand accused of immoral practices in getting babies on to the bottle in all parts of the world. Baby Milk Action say that their tactics range from advertising and misinformation to sending sales reps into hospitals to promote their products in contravention of the International Code.

Seven billion dollars' worth of baby milk is sold across the world each year, and Nestlé sells 50 per cent of the total. A boycott of Nestlé's products has been stepped up in recent years. The pro-breastfeeding movement is backed by WHO, Save the Children, Oxfam, UNICEF and many members of the Church of England Synod.

Breastfeeding in the UK: the way forward

Breastfeeding in Britain is in a very poor state. We now have one of the lowest rates of breastfeeding in Europe. Sixty-five per cent of women begin breastfeeding, but after four months the numbers have dwindled to 25 per cent.

By the time their babies are six weeks old, almost half of British mothers (40 per cent) who started by breastfeeding have turned at least partially to bottles of formula milk. The number of babies being fed on formula milk at four months has almost doubled since 1985, despite mounting research which shows its inadequacy. This is very sad for us, too. As one mother put it:

> I do increasingly think that breastfeeding is a much more important issue than most people believe. There is a terrible devaluation of anything female. To undermine breastfeeding is to undermine everything womanly. It makes you feel you are not doing anything valuable. Yet if you went to a chemist shop and asked them to make a phial of what we can make with our breasts, it would cost a fortune. Breastfeeding can make you feel tremendously proud, tremendously satisfied. But men have tried to take over the process and reproduce it mechanically.

In the late 1980s the government set up the Joint Breastfeeding Initiative to increase the numbers of women breastfeeding after six weeks. Says Dora Henschel, Coordinator of the JBI:

> The government have supported breastfeeding, but there is a lot more to be done. Doctors in particular need to be educated. Many doctors are very ignorant and uninterested in breastfeeding. We have a voluntary agreement with the baby-milk manufacturers – rather than the full WHO code – but it doesn't go far enough. [EC legislation is set to change this soon.]

> We also need to raise the profile of breastfeeding. You don't see it on TV or in the media. You see people making love or giving birth, but not breastfeeding. It would be nice if the TV soaps, if well-known people, talked about it in a positive way. Currently, it's still taboo.

Sheila Kitzinger believes that the most important thing women can do to promote breastfeeding is to feed publicly, and especially in front of children. She also points to the absence of breastfeeding in children's books. Education in schools, of boys as well as girls, is a must.

Chloe Fisher, too, believes that the way forward is through awareness of just how precious breastfeeding is:

> Breastfeeding is an incredible ecological resource, and it costs such a little. In other societies, babies are dying for lack of it. We have to realize that we have done the most horrendous harm in the name of science.

Sally Inch, a midwife and breastfeeding expert, believes there are three hurdles which we have to overcome:

> We need a major change in the attitude of society to breasts and breastfeeding. I think page three has a lot to answer for. Secondly, we need education for health professionals who are still handicapped by textbooks full of rubbish. Many midwives still believe it is helpful to limit feeds and/or sucking time. Sixty per cent of hospitals still give water or a glucose solution to babies although we know this is one of the major contributors to breastfeeding failure.
>
> Thirdly, because of staff cutbacks and the fragmentation of care, there is insufficient opportunity for midwives to learn new skills. If you are the only one on a ward with forty mothers, you can't possibly help women properly. And because women are sent home after forty-eight hours you never learn how they get on, you get no feedback to your advice. The only way is to learn from mothers.

Sally Inch also points out that no one makes any money out of breastfeeding – in contrast to formula milk. The government spends around £40–50,000 a year on promoting breastfeeding, while the formula manufacturers have an advertising budget of £10 million. Yet there is a considerable amount of money – in terms of health care – to be saved through breastfeeding. If all those babies who needed to be hospitalized for gastro-enteritis (up to ten times as many bottle-fed babies suffer from it) were kept out of hospital, the savings would be enormous.

The financial pros and cons of breastfeeding may sway governments: the true benefits of breastfeeding are immeasurable.

5
Making breastfeeding work

This chapter gives the practical information women need about breastfeeding if they are to make an informed choice in feeding their babies.

It is often said that the pro-breastfeeding lobby are at fault in making women who don't breastfeed feel guilty. Mary Renfrew, director of the Midwifery Research Programme at the National Perinatal Epidemiology Unit, is aware of the incalculable benefits of breastfeeding, and she puts it differently:

> If we *don't* persuade women to breastfeed they will feel guilty.

Easier said than fed

Just as we don't often see other women's breasts, many new mothers have never watched another woman breastfeeding. Yet breastfeeding is not an instinct: it is a process which every new mother has to learn for herself, and learn at a time when she is often mentally and physically exhausted.

Yet the physical realities of breastfeeding are difficult for Western women, who are under such pressure to see their breasts as sexual objects. The idea of using them for feeding a baby may be emotionally confusing, and she may even be shy of handling her own breasts. When her new baby starts to suckle with surprising depth she may be disturbed by the animal nature of the experience.

These are all reasons for experiencing anxiety, embarrassment, even fear – feelings which can have an effect on the speed of developing the physical skill of breastfeeding. Gabrielle Palmer suggests we compare learning to breastfeed (as it is done in many modern hospitals) with another sensitive process which involves both psyche and body – making love for the first time:

> Imagine taking the young man to a special sex centre where 'experts' will supervise and instruct him. Assume his partner is equally inexperienced and that he is told to *try* to achieve an erection. As he starts, an 'expert' (who may never have done it himself) watches, criticizes, prods and pulls him about. By the bed is an artificial penis, there in case 'you can't manage it'.

It would take a triumph of concentration and determination on the young man's part if he did 'manage it', just as it takes tremendous perseverance in many women to carry on with breastfeeding in comparable circumstances.

How it happens

In pregnancy, the breasts have already enlarged considerably in readiness for producing milk. Some women have nipples which don't protrude; these are called 'inverted nipples'. However it is not ultimately the nipple shape that matters, but whether the baby can form an adequate 'teat' from the nipple and breast together.

After childbirth, the sensitivity of nipples is increased, and during breastfeeding, the nipples will become erect – just as they do during sex. In pregnancy, too, the Montgomery's tubercles on the areola have become more active, ready to do their job of secreting the lubricating fluid which keeps the nipple soft and supple during suckling.

In late pregnancy the complex of hormones which control milk production start manufacturing colostrum, the yellowish liquid which is the baby's first food. Colostrum is highly nutritious, allowing both mother and baby to rest after the hard work of birth.

After birth, and when the placenta has gone, the mother's oestrogen levels drop quickly and the hormone prolactin gets to work. Prolactin is released in response to the suckling of the baby and when it reaches the network of blood vessels surrounding the milk-producing cells of the breast, milk is created. The more the baby suckles, the more prolactin is released and the more milk is made.

In this way the baby controls the whole process, ensuring that enough milk is produced to meet its needs – provided it is allowed to suckle on the breast whenever it wants to. Prolactin also suppresses ovulation in a fully breastfeeding woman, making breastfeeding the most widespread natural contraceptive around the world. [The term *fully* breastfeeding involves the baby having no other food or drink and at least six feeds a day. However, an additional form of contraception should always be used.]

The baby's suckling also stimulates another hormone – oxytocin – which makes the muscle cells around the milk glands contract. This process – often felt as a strong tingling in the breasts – is called the let-down reflex. It can be so powerful that jets of milk can spray out for several feet. As it happens in both breasts at once, breastfeeding women can stop the milk flow in the breast not being suckled by pressing firmly on the nipple.

The baby's suckling is not the only way of initiating the let-down reflex. Often just the sound or even the sight of her baby can cause the milk to spurt from a mother's nipples in readiness for a feed.

Oxytocin, too, is a hormone with a range of effects. It is sometimes called the 'love' hormone because it also plays a role in orgasm and sexual arousal. Some women describe the let-down reflex as 'something between an orgasm and a sneeze'. Oxytocin may also cause milk to spurt from the breasts during orgasm, reminding us – however uncomfortable we may be with the idea – that sex and breastfeeding are linked in fundamental physical ways.

Successful breastfeeding

Physical inability to breastfeed is very rare. In communities where there is no alternative but to breastfeed, only about one in a hundred women is unable to do so. The World Health Organization now accepts that 97 per cent of women are capable of breastfeeding their babies successfully.

There are two processes involved in getting the milk to the baby. One depends on the active expulsion of milk by the mother in the let-down reflex. The second is the active removal of milk by the baby, using its jaw and tongue. For this to work well, the baby must be properly positioned on the breast so that it can lap the breast tissue into its mouth and 'strip' the milk in a rolling action of its tongue – which is rather like the action of milking a cow by hand.

The key to breastfeeding does not depend on our making milk, as so many of us assume, but on the efficient removal of that milk by the baby.

According to *Successful Breastfeeding*, a handbook by the Royal College of Midwives (RCM):

> If the baby is correctly attached, there should be no friction of the tongue or gums on the nipple, and no movement of breast tissue in and out of the baby's mouth. Thus the baby's sucking should not traumatize the nipple and there should be no soreness.

Pain is a signal that something is going wrong – probably that the baby needs to be repositioned – and if the pain is ignored, the result is often damage to the nipple.

The RCM also recommends that babies should be fed when they want for as long as they want: this is the only way to make sure that a baby is getting what it needs.

Helpful tips

- Feed the baby as soon as possible after birth.
- Feed the baby when it wants, for as long as it wants.
- Feed during the nights as during the day.
- Keep the baby by your bed, or in your bed, from birth onwards.
- Refuse offers of bottles of glucose, formula or water for the baby; these are often given to newborn babies in hospital,

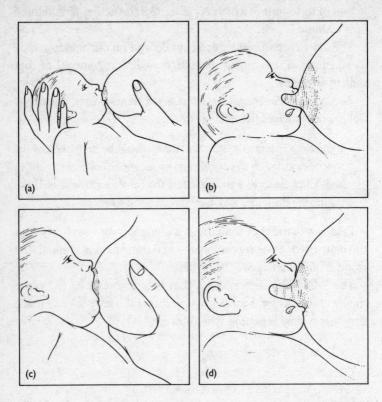

Figure 1: Figures 1(a) and (b) illustrate incorrect positioning. Figures 1(c) and (d) illustrate correct positioning. Source: *Successful Breastfeeding*, Royal College of Midwives

and can undermine breastfeeding. Breastfed babies do not need extra water, even in hot weather.

- To achieve correct positioning:
  1. The baby should face the breast.
  2. The baby should be moved towards the breast: the

nipple is not a bottle teat to be 'put in' the baby's mouth.

3. Let the baby's lips brush against the nipple to encourage the baby to open its mouth wide with tongue down and forwards.

4. As the baby opens its mouth wide, aim the baby's lower lip well below the nipple to ensure that the baby's tongue is in contact with the breast and not just the nipple.

Unhelpful myths

- 'Breastfeeding must be restricted to avoid nipple damage.'
  This idea dates from 'expert advice' at the turn of the century which regarded the nipple as similar to a bottle teat and therefore subject to severe wear and tear.
- 'Feeds should be restricted.'
  This also dates from an 'expert' misconception that over-feeding causes digestive disorders in babies.
- 'Feeds should be stopped after a certain time.'
  Babies take milk from the breast at their own speed, but if left to feed as long as they want to, they will take roughly the same amount of milk as each other.
- 'Feeds should be regularly spaced.'
  Some babies will want to feed at intervals of an hour and a half, whereas others will be happy to wait four to six hours for a feed.

The composition of milk

Breast milk is rather like blood but without the red blood cells, according to Janet Balaskas and Yehudi Gordon in *The Encyclopedia of Pregnancy and Birth*. It has protective white blood cells (leucocytes) to defend against infection and disease, as well as antibodies, enzymes, hormones and other active cells.

Our milk is unique to our species. It is low in protein – because we grow more slowly than other species. It is high in sugar (lactose) to help develop our relatively large brains. Cow's milk – which we often give to human babies instead of our own – is designed to suit calves who need less sugar and more protein than we do. Formula (artificial milk) manufacturers do try to make cow's milk as much like human milk as they can – by diluting it, adding sugar and so on – but breast milk cannot be artificially reproduced.

Even the composition of breast milk – and its flow – will change, according to the stage of the baby's feed, or to the time of day. Mothers who have premature babies will temporarily produce milk which is different in composition from the milk of mothers with full-term babies, and which is ideal for their newborns.

After the colostrum (the highly nutritious fluid provided by the breast in the first few days after birth) comes a transitional phase when the breasts start to make thinner, more watery milk. And then, after about two weeks, the breasts are producing 'mature' milk. Whenever the baby starts to suckle, the 'foremilk' (low fat/high volume) is the first third of her feed. Meanwhile the suckling stimulates the let-down process and the 'hind milk' (high fat/low volume) descends towards the nipple.

Adopting mothers can breastfeed

Most of us assume that milk is produced in our breasts only after babies are born. But the truth is that most women – whether they have given birth or not – can produce milk. Sometimes the sucking of the breasts during sex can cause milk to be produced. There are also reports that men's breasts can produce milk.

In Western societies, adopting mothers have breastfed their new babies, even though they may never have given birth. Some have used a device called a 'Lact-aid' which carries artificial baby milk through a tube into the baby's mouth while she suckles on the breast. Gabrielle Palmer tells the story of a woman who shared the feeding of an adopted child with her sister (who had recently given birth), so that the adopted baby learned to feed on the 'full' breast while gradually stimulating his adoptive mother's breasts to produce milk.

Additionally, there may be a role for drugs such as Domperidone, which can in some circumstances boost the natural production of prolactin to allow breastfeeding. Over a thousand babies under the age of one are adopted every year in Britain, but adoption agencies rarely mention that breastfeeding is a possibility.

Whether women have given birth to their babies or have adopted them, learning to breastfeed can bring inestimable gifts to mothers and babies alike. Babies benefit enormously in terms of physical and emotional health. Women, too, stand to gain in confidence, satisfaction and love. In the most profound sense, we are all the richer when breastfeeding works.

6
Breasts and sex

In physical terms, our breasts have two major functions; maternal and sexual. We have looked at the maternal function in the last two chapters. This chapter looks at the role of breasts in sexual attraction and pleasure.

Frontal globes?

The zoologist Desmond Morris has popularized the theory that human breasts evolved as a kind of erotic buttock substitute once *Homo sapiens* had taken to standing upright:

> If the female of our species was going to successfully shift the interest of the male around to the front, evolution would have to do something to make the frontal region more stimulating. At some point, back in our ancestry, we must have been using the rear approach ... Can we, if we look at the frontal regions of the females of our species, see any structures that might possibly be mimics of the ancient genital display of hemispherical buttocks, and red labia? The answer stands out as clearly as the female bosom itself. The protuberant, hemispherical breasts of the female

must surely be copies of the fleshy buttocks, and the sharply defined red lips around the mouth must be copies of the red labia.

Morris may be right; or he may not. The fact remains that Western men today (and he is one of them) tend to perceive the breasts primarily as a spur to sex and an organ of pleasure. Caressing and sucking of breasts and nipples can be intensely pleasurable aspects of sex for both men and women.

Women's pleasure

In *The Hite Report on Female Sexuality* (1976), women describe their experience of sexual arousal in terms of sensations all over the body, including the breasts:

> There is an exquisite tension, an ache, a hunger – and my breasts get tight and feel as if they must be touched.

> A rush – hot – yearning in my breasts to be touched . . .

> A heightened sensitivity all over, a vaguely burning sensation in the clitoral area, and a sort of yearning to be touched on my breasts . . .

Touching of breasts also plays a part in women's sexual fantasies:

> I used to have a recurring fantasy that I was a gym teacher and had a classful of girls standing in front of me, nude. I went up and down the rows feeling all their breasts and getting a lot of pleasure out of it. When I first had this fantasy at thirteen I was ashamed. I

> thought that something was wrong with me. Now I can enjoy it
> because I feel it's okay to enjoy other women's bodies. (*Our Bodies,
> Ourselves*, Angela Phillips and Jill Rakusen)

Some women's breasts are so sexually sensitive that their owners can reach orgasm through touching of their breasts alone. Others find quite the opposite – that touching of their breasts is irritating or simply boring. Neither response is 'normal' or 'abnormal': women's sexual response is as individual and varied as we are, and can change over time.

In a survey of women for their book *The Breast*, Drs Penny and Andrew Stanway found that:

- Seventeen per cent claimed they could experience an orgasm through breast-play alone.
- Seventy per cent said their breasts' sensitivity changed with the monthly cycle, becoming tender and painful at times.
- Half of women said they played with their own breasts as part of masturbation. One in twenty said they sucked their own nipples.
- Women most like to have their breasts kissed and stroked during sex. They were not so keen on breast squeezing – which was more popular as a practice with men.
- A third of women find other women's breasts sexually exciting, and are 'turned on' by pictures in soft-porn magazines. (Nearly half thought the material was harmful, misleading or disgusting.)
- Sixty-four per cent of women said they had found breastfeeding 'sexually pleasant' or 'sensual'. Half of women found their sexual relationship didn't change at all during breastfeeding, despite a common worry that their partners would 'go off them'.

Men's pleasure

In *The Hite Report on Male Sexuality* (1981), Shere Hite asked men, 'What things about women do you most admire?' Their responses were mostly in terms of women's physical characteristics, or parts of the body that they liked. Many replies mentioned breasts:

> I enjoy very much looking at attractive women. I especially enjoy it if they are bra-less.

> I like women who are just plain soft and cuddly. I love breasts of course, but I'm even more turned on by nipples. They're like little penises.

> I like a woman's ass and tits.

> Nice legs are much more attractive to me than breasts. More girls have good legs than good breasts; and good is not equivalent to huge. Big tits are as unaesthetic as thick thighs; small-breasted girls are not losers either. But breasts that are of size and shape proportionate to the girl's general physique are relatively rare; they do draw the eye and invite the hand. The right-sized breast is one that fits a man's hand.

Shere Hite points out that these men sound as if they own women's bodies, discussing their merits and demerits as they might discuss a car. Breasts of a particular type were high on the list of consumer demand:

> Breasts not too small or too large with pronounced areolas.

> A woman should be not more than five foot five approaching the 36–24–36 numbers or exceeding them (breasts only, as long as they don't hang).

I like women's breasts, but I prefer that they not be too large. When they hang down into her armpits when she's supine is too large.

I like moderate-sized boobs on ladies. I don't like the model, flat-chested look, but I don't like cow udders either.

I don't like droopy breasts. You can be top heavy and sag and look attractive. But saggy breasts are unappealing sexually.

As we know, firm breasts generally mean young breasts, and behind many of these remarks is an unabashed ageism. Often the ageism is combined with a staggering double standard, as in this statement from a 53-year-old man:

I am definitely attracted to younger women and repelled by older ones. Why? The young ones have fresh, beautifully formed bodies with firm flesh and skin, and the older ones are not nearly so attractive. Wrinkles and sagging breasts repel me.

From a woman's point of view, age makes no difference to sexual pleasure in our breasts. We have the same potential to feel pleasure from our breasts whether young or old, firm or soft, throughout our lives.

In the laboratory

Sexologists have measured what physically happens to breasts during sex. In the early 'excitement' phase of arousal, the tiny muscles of the nipple will contract to make them erect. This happens in some men, as well as women.

The nipples can also grow longer (by up to half an inch) and wider (by as much as a quarter of an inch) as blood collects in and around them. The pattern of veins on the breasts may become more noticeable, and the breasts grow larger – by as much as a third more than their usual size, particularly in women who haven't breastfed. (Women who have breastfed have a more developed system of veins to drain the blood away.) The areolae also swell and the breasts may become covered with the 'sex flush', a red flush which may look like a rash.

Then comes the 'plateau' phase of arousal, in which the breasts become more swollen, followed (sometimes) by orgasm. After orgasm, the whole process goes into reverse, with breasts and areolae returning to normal in the 'resolution' phase. After this, many women find they don't want their breasts touched for some time, although some women can return to the excitement phase again and continue on to another orgasm.

Researchers have found that lesbian couples usually spend much more time and care on breast play than heterosexual couples. In their study Masters and Johnson found that:

> The full breast was always stimulated manually and orally (by the same sex partner) with particular concentration focused on the nipples. Interestingly, almost scrupulous care was taken by the stimulator to spend an equal amount of time with each breast. As much as ten minutes were sometimes spent in intermittent breast stimulation before genital play was introduced.

Masters and Johnson also noted that the lesbian caressing her partner's breasts seems to do so with

> more attention to her partner's responses, while men often approach heterosexual breast stimulation more for their own arousal than for their partner's pleasure.

Lesbian lovers, they found, seem more aware of the fact that breast touching can be painful just before a period, 'while many men seem oblivious to this fact'.

Gay men also use nipple stimulation – manual and oral – in their early sexual touching, which, say Masters and Johnson, almost invariably leads to an erection for the man stimulated. Interestingly, they found that few wives stimulate their husband's nipples as part of sex play.

Sexual feelings and breastfeeding

Then there is the vexed question of breastfeeding and sex. In total contrast to the close association between 'breasts and sex', 'breast*feeding* and sex' are not supposed to go together. They are the oil and water of sexual morality; they are cultural chalk and cheese.

Despite all we hear of the joys of motherhood, there is deep and meaningful silence about the sensual or sexual pleasure which can accompany breastfeeding. This is a taboo subject, too confusingly near our fears of incest for comfort (see Chapter Four). But what are the physical implications of sex in the months when we are still breastfeeding?

Many women – and men – lose the desire for sex while women are breastfeeding, and some couples go through months, or even years, when sex is no longer part of the agenda. This can be deeply upsetting and disappointing, usually for the male partner, and especially so when the couple had no prior warning that this might happen.

Yet there are good physiological and psychological reasons for the woman's loss of interest in sex while breastfeeding. She is likely to be quite exhausted for a start, which is never good for sex, and it could be that the hormone prolactin – released while breastfeeding – is acting to inhibit the libido.

However, other couples find that the breastfeeding months are more erotic than ever before. For a start, the breasts are usually quite a lot bigger, which can be a bonus. There can also be a new level of freedom from worries about contraception (if women are *fully* breastfeeding) which allows more spontaneity.

Some men also enjoy the fact that their partner's breasts are producing milk and may want to taste the milk. Although there is a myth that such men are 'robbing' the baby's milk supply, it can do no harm at all for a man to drink at the same source. Because the breasts work on a supply-and-demand basis, more milk will be produced to make up for what has been taken.

Some women also find that breastfeeding itself is pleasurable and these feelings can vary from mildly sensual to extremely erotic. These feelings are perfectly natural.

For some couples then, the breastfeeding time is a time to take a holiday from sex. But for others, it is a time to enjoy breasts and a woman's sexuality in a deeper way than ever before.

7
The well breast

Not many of us know how breasts work, which makes it hard to be confident that our own breasts are healthy and normal. This chapter describes how the well breast develops and changes, from month to month as well as throughout our lives, and explains how to look after your breasts.

But the issue which preoccupies many women (in part because it preoccupies so many men) is that of breast size.

Breasts big and small

It is a common assumption that the bigger a woman's breasts, the 'sexier' she is. In reality, breast size makes no difference to a woman's capacity to receive pleasure from sex, nor to her desire for sex. Breast size makes no difference to a woman's ability to breastfeed either.

Girls' breasts develop at different ages. But generally, the breasts have reached their full size by around the age of seventeen. The size of our breasts depends on how much fat our bodies have deposited there, and on how much glandular tissue we have. Both of these are influenced by our genetic inheritance – which comes from our fathers as much as from our mothers. Fatter women tend to have larger breasts, and women who diet often notice that the first part of their bodies to shrink is their breasts.

Many of us have one breast which is slightly larger than the other. Some women buy two different-sized bras and re-stitch them to fit unequal breasts. Others have one breast which is significantly bigger. This can happen in women who do repetitive jobs with one hand which develop their chest muscle on one side, or it can happen when one of the breasts doesn't develop.

If, however, you suddenly find that one of your breasts has become bigger than the other, you may be developing an infection, a cyst or another health problem (perhaps cancer), so *do* go to see your doctor.

There are also wide and natural variations in the positioning of women's breasts. Some are low-down, others high-up. The position of the nipple on the breast varies too, as does the size of the areola, which can be anything from one to four inches in diameter.

The developing breast

Throughout a woman's life, her breasts are frequently changing. They change rapidly with puberty. They change every month with the hormones of the menstrual cycle. They change with pregnancy, again with breastfeeding, again with menopause and again with ageing. They change so often that only by becoming familiar with our own breasts, month by month, can we know what is normal and healthy for us.

This long process of change begins in the six-week-old foetus when a number of embryonic nipples (or papillae) develop along the two 'milk lines' that run from armpit to groin. This happens in both male and female foetuses.

By nine weeks into a pregnancy, most of the milk line has disappeared leaving just one nipple on either side of the chest. Soon the nipple bud develops together with milk ducts and a collecting reservoir. Pigment forms around the nipple to make the areola. This phase of development now comes to a halt, and for females there won't be further significant changes until puberty.

Sometimes babies are born with extra nipples which show up anywhere along the milk line and can look like little warts or nipples. These are more common in men, but they have the potential to develop into extra breasts in women. In the Middle Ages, according to Drs Andrew and Penny Stanway people believed that extra nipples were for feeding the familiar spirits of witches – and so they burnt these unlucky women at the stake.

Not much happens to our breasts in childhood, but as soon as the hormones of puberty swing into action, the breasts start growing – and at a much faster rate than the rest of the body. In the earliest stages of breast growth, a small mound of tissue – the 'breast bud' – appears. Gradually, the nipple and areola enlarge and the contour of the breast becomes more prominent.

This growth of the breasts is known as the 'thelarche' and it is usually the first sign of puberty, beginning as early as the age of eight and up to about the age of thirteen. The duct system gradually develops in the breasts and fat is deposited, making the breasts larger. Some girls will develop large breasts very quickly. Others will always have small breasts.

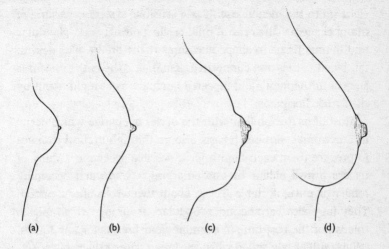

Figure 2: The stages of breast development at puberty. (a) Breast bud elevation; (b) growth and protrusion of the nipple; (c) elevation of the secondary areolar mound; (d) regression of the areolar mound to the level of the general breast contour. Source: Hughes, L.E., Mansel, R.E. and Webster D., *Benign Disorders and Diseases of the Breast*, Baillière Tindall, 1989

The adult breast

With all of today's emphasis on breasts as sex symbols, it's easy to forget that they are designed chiefly as working organs. That work is feeding babies, but most of today's breasts are out of a job for most of the time – with implications explored in the next chapter.

The changes of puberty have developed a complete milk-production system, which is in a continual state of readiness right up to the menopause. It is a sensitive system consisting of many elements (the central milk-production network, glandular and fibrous tissue to shape and support the breast, plus nerves, fat, blood vessels and connective tissue), and the entire system is subject to the many and repeated fluctuations brought about by the female hormones.

Most of us are familiar with the cycles of change which occur in our wombs. But our breasts also go through cyclical changes to prepare them each month for a possible pregnancy. Many of us are aware of our breasts enlarging – and often becoming tender or uncomfortable – from about two weeks after a period. They may also become more 'nodular' or lumpy, which means this is not the best time to examine your breasts for any lumps. (Wait until after a period when the breasts are at their softest.)

Breasts are thought to be at their most sensitive to touch at ovulation – halfway through the cycle – and at the time of your period. (Women on the Pill will not experience this peak at ovulation.) Breasts will stay enlarged until three or four days into a period and then return to their 'normal' size.

We don't understand the details of how breasts enlarge, but it seems that fluid retention in the whole of the breast makes them tense and sensitive at particular times. Most women's breasts will increase in size by up to a third with extra fluid together with an increased blood flow. (Women on the Pill generally have less swelling.) If no pregnancy follows, the fluids and accumulated tissues are broken down by cells in the lymph system and drained from the breast into the body.

Cyclical breast change

Virtually every woman gets some kind of different breast sensation just before a period. Some women feel pain in both breasts,
which varies with their menstrual cycle. This is rarely a sign of
any other breast problem, but if you want to end the pain there
are various things you can do which are outlined in the next
chapter. (If you are on the Pill or HRT, or your periods are just
beginning or ending, you will not be ovulating and so won't
have this kind of breast discomfort.)

If your cycle ends in pregnancy, there will be profound changes
in the size of the breast as well as its structure and function. The
breasts of pregnant women can double in size as breast tissue
increases, milk ducts develop, new blood vessels form and blood
flow increases by up to 180 per cent.

These many breast changes go on year in and year out until
the menopause eventually brings an end to the constant flux of
female hormones. For about ten years after the age of thirty-five,
the glandular tissue of the breast slowly shrinks, to be replaced
by fat. From forty-five onwards, the glandular tissue disappears
at a faster rate while more fat and connective tissue is laid down.
Later still, the fat may shrink away, giving the characteristically
soft, pendulous shape to the breasts of older women. Age makes
little difference, however, when it comes to the sexual pleasure a
woman can enjoy from her breasts and her nipples.

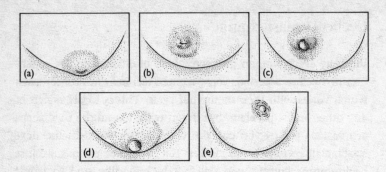

Figure 3: It is normal for the size and shape of nipples to vary greatly from woman to woman. Nipples may be prominent, flat or inverted.

Nipples and areolae

Like breasts, nipples and areolae normally come in all sorts of shapes and sizes. They vary in colour from pale pink to black – depending on a woman's skin colour. During her first pregnancy, a woman's nipples and areolae will become darker – and stay that way. The Pill can make the nipple area darker too.

Nipples can also change their shape, protruding from the cone of the breast when their many small muscles contract to make them erect. This can happen in response to cold weather, the friction of clothes, sexual stimulation and/or breastfeeding. But not all nipples protrude. Inverted nipples are common in children and in men. Some mature women have grown up with inverted nipples, which stay inverted. But if a nipple should turn inwards in adulthood, get your breast checked by a doctor.

The skin of the nipple and the areola is hairless, but some women do have quite long hairs which grow around the areola.

Sometimes hairs will grow as a result of the hormones of pregnancy, or because of changes in the use of the Pill. Women who don't like the look of these hairs can pluck them out without doing any harm.

The areola has special sweat glands called Montgomery's tubercles, which also enlarge during pregnancy. Their job is to secrete a lubricant called 'sebum' which protects and softens the nipple during breastfeeding. The tip of the nipple itself has ten to fifteen deep fissures which provide the outlets for the milk ducts.

While the skin of the breast is very much like the skin of the rest of the body, the skin of the nipple has an especially rich supply of nerve endings, making it a powerfully erogenous zone. Sexual stimulation and breastfeeding will both cause blood to flow strongly to the breast, making breast and nipple swell considerably.

Some discharge from the nipple is common, even if you are not breastfeeding or have not done so for years. But don't make a habit of squeezing your nipples; you could do yourself damage. (See Chapter Nine for more information on nipple discharge.)

Inside the breast

The insides of our breasts look rather like clusters of grapes. Each breast has about twenty grape-like lobes, where milk is made. Each lobe has many tiny lobules which secrete milk into the lobe. Milk ducts lead from each lobe and gather at the nipple. These ducts are like the stalks of the bunch of grapes.

The breast lobes are separated and supported in a bed of

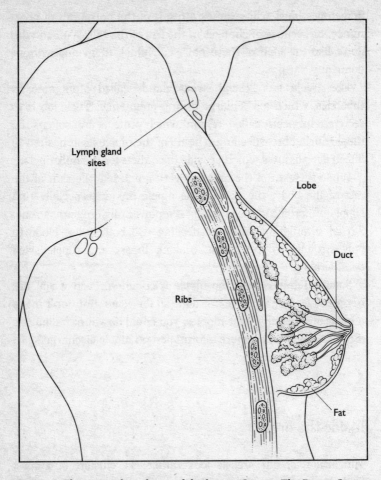

Figure 4: The internal workings of the breast. Source: The Breast Cancer Digest, US, DHEW, Publication No. 79–1691

connective and fibrous tissue. The average weight of a breast is about seven ounces, while the average weight of a breast which is producing milk is some seventeen ounces. All this weight is carried by suspensory ligaments, or fibrous bands, which connect the skin of the breasts to the upper chest wall. These bands do weaken and stretch over time.

There is no muscle in the breast, apart from the tiny muscles around the milk ducks and the nipple. This means that you cannot build up the shape or size of the breast itself by doing exercises. However, it *is* possible to do exercises which will build up the muscles of the chest wall *under* the breast – which will in turn push the breast forward, making it look bigger.

If you are young and you have small breasts, it is quite possible to go bra-less without any long term ill-effects on your body. But in larger-breasted women gravity will probably take its toll over the years and unsupported breasts will tend to sag earlier. You may feel this is important, but equally, you may not. In any case, our breasts do tend to naturally sink down and become flatter as we get older. In some other cultures this pendulous shape is considered more attractive than the high-up, teenage shape emphasized so strongly in the West.

Breast care

Charlene Bargeron of the Breast Care Campaign proposes a new dinner-party game for the 1990s: 'Name Your Breast Lumps'. Over the after-dinner mints, the relaxed, modern woman will be practising a swift self-exam – 'Ah, here's Roger, back again already! And Fred too! Well, it is coming up to that time of the month.'

Charlene is only half joking, because – at the very least – we need a new and positive approach to our own breast health.

Unfortunately for women, there has been a lot of muddle about the issue of breast self-examination in recent years. For a while the orthodoxy was that we *should* all do regular BSE (breast self-examination). Health books and women's magazines showed women lying on their backs, breasts dotted with arrows, palms of the hand following those arrows in a systematic search-and-destroy mission. For most of us who hardly ever did it, BSE seemed like just something else we ought to be finding time to do, something else to feel guilty about.

Then, the government's Chief Medical Officer, Sir Donald Acheson, caused a big stir on the eve of his retirement by suggesting that BSE was all a waste of time. He made the undisputed point that by the time a cancer is big enough to be felt by a woman's fingers, there is little that medicine can do to 'cure' her.

The Department of Health initially backed him by confirming that there is no proof that self-exam reduces the death rate from breast cancer. It made the further point that BSE can have negative effects in increasing anxiety amongst women. A far more 'scientific' way was for women to attend regular NHS breast screenings.

This U-turn in official medical advice caused an uproar. It was as if the emperor himself had admitted to wearing no clothes. But when the uproar died down, some common-sense voices emerged to argue that the emperor had missed the point.

Better than nothing?

Many health professionals and women's health groups said that
self-exam may not detect cancer early, but it was better than
nothing. After all, only those of us over fifty are eligible for
screening, whereas about a quarter of breast cancers turn up in
women under fifty.

Breast cancer charities also pointed out that thousands of
women who have been effectively treated for breast cancer first
noticed the disease in themselves. Mr Ian Fentiman, an eminent
surgeon, was quoted by the medical press as saying that '90 per
cent of the lumps discovered, women find for themselves, so to
suggest that they should stop self-examination is ridiculous'
(*Pulse*, 21.9.91).

The government quickly came out with new guidelines. 'Breast
Awareness' was the new way forward (although not to be relied
upon as a primary screening method), and women should make
a habit of checking their breasts for any lumps and changes.
Most of us said, 'What's the difference?', and carried on neglect-
ing to check ourselves anyway. (Only about one in five British
women regularly checks herself.)

It remains true that in their early stages most cancers are too
small for you to detect yourself. But there are still some very
good reasons for us all to get to know our breasts.

Good reasons to know your breasts

By touching and looking at our own breasts, we demystify them,
we become comfortable with them. At the same time, we are
gaining knowledge about our bodies, and that knowledge is
power. In a culture that tells us our breasts belong to men (and
occasionally to children), we are laying claim to them again as
well as dismissing old notions that it's 'dirty' to 'touch ourselves'.
And in looking after our breasts we are taking care of ourselves
– a bold thing in itself for some women who are expected to take
care of everybody *but* themselves.

In practical terms, too, there are still good reasons for getting
to know your breasts. Once you know what they feel like and
how they change, you are far less likely to feel that awful surge
of panic as you suddenly notice they have gone all lumpy. And if
you are going to find a lump that turns out to be cancer, the
sooner you find it the better. It could mean less surgery than if it
was found later; a lumpectomy perhaps, rather than a
mastectomy.

According to Dr Pat Last, consultant in women's health to
BUPA Health Services, some cancers which can be felt as lumps
do not even show up on mammograms.

Furthermore, because screening is only done every three years,
a percentage of new breast cancers will be detectable by self-
exam before they ever get to a mammogram.

When to examine?

Monthly if you can, but every few months is better than not at all. The main thing is to do it at the same point in your cycle so you know what your breasts normally feel like at that time. Also, choose one method of checking your breasts which best suits you – and stick to it. That way you can continue to compare like with like.

A good time to check your breasts is when they are at their least lumpy – which is in the week or two after your period, before you ovulate.

If you have passed the menopause, your breasts won't be changing with a monthly cycle any more, but it helps to remind yourself with a regular date – like the first of the month. If you are having HRT, the best time to check your breasts is when you've finished a cycle of hormones.

How to check your breasts

Many of us never really look at our breasts. So take a few minutes when getting undressed one evening: stand in front of the mirror, raise your hands above your head and get acquainted with your own unique shape, size and quirks.

Once you know what your breasts normally look like, you will be able to keep an eye out for any of the following:

- An unusual change in the outline, shape or size.
- Puckering or dimpling of the skin.

- A lump or thickening in the breast or armpit, which is persistent, unchanging through your cycle and probably at least half an inch across.
- Any flaking of your skin or discharge from the nipple.

Next, lie down in the bath or on your bed, and feel one breast at a time, using your right hand to examine your left breast and vice versa. There are various ways of doing this – working in a spiral, or in sections, or as if along the spokes of a wheel. It doesn't matter which method you choose, as long as you use the same method each time.

Use the flat of your fingers, as if your hand is an iron and you are 'ironing' your breast. Remember that breast tissue extends up to the armpit and nearly to the collar-bone, so feel these areas too.

If you are aged between fifty and sixty-five you can also take advantage of the national breast-screening programme which will automatically call you for a mammogram every three years. And if you are over sixty-five, you can still ask to be screened. The actual process of X-ray is not painful. But to take the 'picture', your breasts are squashed between an X-ray plate and a plastic plate, and some women – especially those with breasts that are larger or smaller than most – find it very uncomfortable.

BUPA offers a useful Breast Screening Video at £9.95 (incl. p & p), from The Marketing Dept, BUPA Medical Centre, 300 Gray's Inn Road, London WC1X 8DU.

Even if you do find a breast lump, nine times out of ten it will be harmless. But don't ignore it: make an appointment with your doctor. Armed with information about how your breasts work, you are well placed to ask the right questions and to understand what your doctor tells you. At the very least you will be better able to cope with the extreme anxiety which so often plagues women when well breasts become unwell breasts.

8
Doctoring breasts:
a women's issue

Sooner or later there comes a point for many of us when self-help and self-examination are no longer enough: we have found a breast lump, or we are plagued by breast pain. The next step – we are advised again and again – is to go to the doctor.

Unfortunately, something is going seriously wrong between many women and their doctors when it comes to breast care. The accounts that women give of their treatments all too often tell of insensitivity and sexism.

There are many reasons behind this failure in care. Some are cultural: we seem to be uniquely ignorant and uncomfortable with breasts in our culture. Others are historical: breast problems have traditionally been dismissed as 'women's problems', i.e. unreal and 'neurotic'. Still others are political: underfunding in our health service often means that doctors have mammoth workloads and insufficient time to respond as women would like them to.

There is also a fundamental gender issue here: it is women who have breast problems, but it is (usually) men who treat breast problems. Many women don't like having to take their tops off and be looked at and prodded by a male doctor. Many doctors don't feel comfortable about it either.

This chapter explores women's experiences with the medical profession when it comes to breasts, beginning with the stories of two women who have had common (benign) breast problems.

Paula: 'Not knowing is the worst thing . . .'

Paula was thirty-three when she first noticed a lump in her breast. She waited two days to make sure she wasn't 'imagining things' and then went to see her GP. A year later she was in good health, but still dismayed and incredulous at the seven stressful months that she had to wait for treatment.

Paula's GP wanted to examine her at least three times before she was referred for further treatment. 'I had to go before a period, during a period, and after a period. In the meantime I lost a stone in weight.' The weight loss was probably because she was so anxious about the outcome, yet in itself it added to the anxiety.

It was five months before Paula was referred to a surgeon at a London hospital. He told her to wait two more months to see if the lump was still there. But after the two months, the lump had not gone and Paula was told 'we need to find out if this is benign or not'.

She was then sent for a scan. For Paula, the experience of the scanning clinic was traumatic in itself: 'You sit all in white robes next to these women who know they have got cancer. Some of them burst into tears when they talk about it, but others are really strong and cracking jokes the whole time.'

After the scan, Paula's consultant rang her surgeon and asked him to come over. 'I'll never forget it,' Paula says. 'I was lying on a couch and the doctors were talking over me. The consultant looked at the scan and said, "Oh, I don't like the look of that at all! That should have come out before now." Of course I thought "I've got cancer, they're going to cut my breast off . . ."'

Paula is full of praise and gratitude for the nursing staff who looked after her at the hospital where her lump was removed.

But she was sent home on the day after the operation, still hardly able to move. She convalesced at her parents' home for ten days before travelling to London to hear the results of her operation: 'When I got there they told me they had lost my records, and I had to go home again.'

She travelled to the hospital a week later only to be told that her records had been lost yet again. But this time her mother had accompanied her and insisted on staying until Paula's records were found.

At last she was told that her breast lump had been benign. Like eleven out of twelve women who seek treatment for a breast disorder, she did not have cancer. Paula was told she had been suffering from 'fibrocystic disease' (see Chapter Nine for more information).

Even now she doesn't fully understand what happened to her: 'They never explained it to me. I found out what I know from a book about fibrocystic disease.'

For Paula, the long wait for information was the worst part of her experience: 'In the end you don't really care if you've got cancer. Not knowing is the worst thing. If I ever had another lump I would not go to my GP, I would go straight to the hospital and demand another scan.'

As for the future, she says that her scar has healed well, but her confidence in treatment for breast disorders hasn't recovered: 'I think I'm all right, but I don't really know . . .'

Sarah: 'I don't trust them enough to go back . . .'

Sarah was in her mid-thirties when she found a small, but very painful lump in her breast: 'I wasn't too worried because I knew the cancerous ones don't move about and aren't usually painful. But because my grandmother died of breast cancer, the thought was at the back of my mind.'

She went to see her GP in Somerset who referred her to a consultant at the local hospital. He confirmed that the lump was a blocked duct, perhaps caused by the mastitis she had suffered when feeding her third child. 'He said it was too small to do anything with, but that there was nothing to worry about,' says Sarah. 'He told me to take evening primrose oil and it should disperse. I found him cold and very unhelpful, and it upset me.'

Yet she did as he suggested, although she found the evening primrose oil was 'very expensive. You can get it on prescription now – but my God – grudgingly!' Then, with a change of contraceptive pill, Sarah found her breasts had become very lumpy and tender: 'I asked for an appointment with a woman GP (our male family doctor's manner is somewhat offhand) and she referred me back to the same consultant.'

By now she was used to the huge waiting room and – after being weighed, giving samples and so on – being called into a room and told, 'Take your top things off'.

'They leave you sitting there for about twenty minutes, topless, with nothing to do or read. You are at such a disadvantage by the time the doctor comes in. Then he stands over you, looking down. I am inhibited by all that. It makes me forget half the things I want to ask, and I don't remember until I'm on my way home. By now I've got wise to it and I don't take my top off until the doctor has come in and has talked to me – with my clothes on.'

Sarah also finds it unnerving that, each time, her doctor would come into the room reading her notes: 'It's so rude. It makes you wonder – do they know why I'm here? And it puts you on the defensive – do they think I shouldn't be here? It makes it hard to have confidence in them.'

This time her consultant referred her for a mammogram, which happened after a further three-month wait. 'That was a very mechanical experience. "Take your top off", no chat, grab. It was ghastly. She had warned me that as I was quite small it might be uncomfortable but I didn't expect her to clamp down quite so hard. The pressure is phenomenal. I couldn't wait to get away.'

The result of the mammogram – eventually relayed by her GP – was 'fine'. But when Sarah's lump got bigger again her GP sent her back to the same clinic: 'I expected to see my usual consultant, but instead his registrar came in – reading my notes – and said, "We can deal with this one, no problems, I'll use a fine needle to take it out." '

He told the nurse to stand by Sarah, and without any anaesthetic (as is usual practice), stuck a needle into her breast: 'I have never experienced anything so painful in my life,' she says. 'It was worse than childbirth. I nearly broke the nurse's hand. Then he said, "That'll be fine, I've got a lot of stuff out", and he disappeared again.

'I was speechless. I had told him the consultant had said it was too small to get out. But there you are, topless, caught. It made me feel quite sick afterwards.

'I did see my consultant again and told him what happened – that it had been the most excruciating experience – but all he said was that I could go back on the evening primrose oil or have surgery.'

By this stage, however, Sarah had lost all confidence: 'I decided I'd rather just live with it. I don't trust them enough to go back. I ignore the lump now. If it gets a knock from the children – you know how they launch themselves at you – it does swim into the back of my mind that I have breast cancer in my family. I would go back to the same woman GP, but not to the hospital: the consultants just don't seem to be that caring.'

Lack of empathy: a UK problem

These two case histories have many elements which women say are typical of breast health care in this country – even of women's health care in general. The waiting, the fear, the lack of communication are common experiences. So is the business of being talked about over our heads, and being expected to wait, semi-clothed, in bare and chilly cubicles.

And when it comes to breasts, these negative experiences seem to be all the more acute. Women remember them for years afterwards much as they remember bad experiences in childbirth. This is because breasts are so important to our sense of self, our psyche, our sexuality. But sadly for us, not all British doctors seem to fully understand what breasts mean to women.

Professor Robert Mansel, a world authority on benign breast disease from the University of Wales College of Medicine, has spent a lifetime talking to women and to GPs about breast health. He believes that:

> In this country, there is a lack of empathy for women with breast problems. It's an emotional issue; we are not tuned in to the problem. In other countries, the place of the breast is regarded as more important. At international conferences held in other countries there is always a lecture on the breast in art, or on the psychosexual aspects of breast disease.

In contrast, the British don't take breasts seriously – except as the location for breast cancer. There are no equivalent conferences, no comparable psychosexual and cultural input. When I asked him for a contact in the psychosexual field who would be able to shed light on breast issues, Professor Mansel couldn't help me. A trawl of psychotherapists and psychosexual journals also drew a blank: it seems that (apart from in the field of cancer) no one has published any papers or done research in the area of breasts.

Our cultural refusal to think seriously about breasts has meant that women with breast disorders often get labelled 'neurotic'. According to Professor Mansel:

> Doctors tend to say that women who sit around all day at home get too introverted and think about themselves too much – and so they go to their GPs complaining of breast problems.

Yet apart from the obvious sexism of such a view, there is plenty of scientific evidence that women with breast problems are no more 'neurotic' than anyone else. When Marks & Spencer ran a screening programme for their employees, they found that nearly half of women staff complained of breast pain. These are hardly women who 'sit at home thinking about themselves'.

Another study from the Cardiff Breast Clinic tried to measure the 'neurosis' in women patients. Doctors found that women complaining of breast pain had no more signs of neurosis than women complaining of varicose veins. In fact, they had marginally less.

Ancient prejudices

There is a long history of prejudice behind such attitudes to 'women's ailments'. Nineteenth-century physicians believed that breast complaints occurred in women with 'irritable', 'nervous' or 'excitable' systems and this idea persists today in the 'neurotic' myth. A major medical textbook which must have influenced many of today's doctors describes women with breast pain as 'frustrated, unhappy nulliparae' (women without children), while another leading authority in the field has described women with breast pain as 'in general, unstable and hypochondriachal, although they are not frankly psychotic'.

The link between premenstrual tension and breast problems has exacerbated medical misunderstanding. Some doctors are quick to slap on the 'neurotic' label when it comes to anything related to women's periods. (The very word 'hysteria' derives from the Greek word for womb.) The American breast surgeon and writer Dr Susan Love observes that the reality of breast pain has been denied, 'just as menstrual pain was denied until ten years ago. [The inference is] it's all psychosomatic, it's all in their heads.'

Professor Mansel, from a UK perspective, has seen the distressing results of that denial on women who suffer from breast pain. Sometimes the pain is so severe that they want their breasts amputated – yet they can't get doctors to take their problem seriously:

> In Britain breast pain is seen as a nuisance. It's a troublesome thing that gets in the way of finding breast cancer. It is regarded as a non-condition, and therefore – the thinking goes – it doesn't need treatment. Doctors are very resistant to treating breast pain. They

say things like, 'I sent her away with a flea in her ear.' Yet they wouldn't say that about the pain of rheumatoid arthritis for example. They think breast pain is a woman's lot.

Men's problem with women's problems

How then do we expect doctors to react to us when we turn up in their surgeries with a breast problem? We can expect them, as professionals, to treat us respectfully, to listen to our concerns and to offer us the best medical advice. But a man doesn't shed all of his cultural attitudes (these have been explored in Chapter Two) when he takes off his coat at the surgery door.

According to one staff member at Breast Cancer Care:

> Young doctors get quite embarrassed about breasts. It's the male/ female thing. They do have to steel themselves to do examinations.

Women patients who perceive a doctor's embarrassment may find it difficult to ask for a breast examination:

> From time to time when I see my GP he says, 'You do examine your breasts don't you?', and I feel that's a hurdle he wants to get quickly over. He's not sure if I want him to examine my breasts, and I feel he doesn't want to do it, so I say, 'They're fine', and on we go from there.

But there are other complex messages about breasts which women say they pick up from their doctors. Another Breast Cancer Care worker has noticed a range of responses in doctors:

> Their responses vary from embarrassment, to fear of litigation, to

perplexity. Doctors often feel at a loss. They don't know what to do for the best about breast pain. There is no consensus about the best treatments for breast cancer either. They don't know how to help us with our 'women's problems' and they don't know how to feel for us.

A fuss about nothing?

Whatever the reasons for a doctor's feelings, and whether the doctor is a man or a woman, much damage to women's confidence in health care is done when doctors react patronizingly or dismissively to women with breast problems. Over and again women say that – having tried to act responsibly by taking 'suspicious' symptoms to a doctor – they are made to feel they are 'making a fuss about nothing' and 'wasting the doctor's valuable time'.

Young women in particular seem to attract a lot of medical scorn, perhaps because doctors know (but women often don't) that their chances of having cancer are very small:

> I thought I had something terrible and went to my doctor. He referred me to a clinic, where they made me strip to the waist and wait for ages in a cold room. When the doctor examined me, he told me I was making a big fuss about nothing. I was made to feel I was wasting the doctor's valuable time. It will be a long time before I go to a doctor again about a breast problem.

> When I was in my early twenties I thought I found a lump and I was referred by my GP to a clinic. The doctor who examined me there was so rude and patronizing that it still makes me furious to

think about it. He spoke to me as if I was a complete idiot and accused me of examining myself by poking my breasts rather than feeling with the flat of my hand. I was utterly humiliated.

Can male doctors do the best job?

Breasts can mean life, femininity, nurture. They can also mean death, illness, cancer. Any health professional dealing with breast disorders cannot be fully effective if he or she is not aware of their deep human implications.

This raises the question: 'Can any male doctor really empathize with a woman who has breast problems?' The American breast surgeon and best-selling author Dr Susan Love seems to think not:

> Even the most sensitive, sympathetic man can't understand a woman's complex emotional relationship to her breasts. [Men] don't know, in their own bodies, what it means to have breasts; they haven't felt that slight adolescent itching as the small bump on the chest grows into a real breast; they haven't set out self-consciously with their mothers to buy a 'training bra'; they haven't fretted over whether a party dress shows too little or too much cleavage. And they haven't faced the nightmare of mastectomy that haunts almost every woman in our culture, and surfaces with even the most harmless breast problem.

Not all women would agree. Some, especially those who have come to trust and respect their family doctors over a long period of time, say they are quite happy to see a man about their breasts. Others have had experience of women doctors who are no more sympathetic than their male colleagues. But the fact remains that many women feel easier about being examined by someone of their own gender, and would go to a woman doctor for breast symptoms much more readily than to a man.

That fact must have implications for health care, and especially for our breast-cancer death rate. There are eminent men in the breast-cancer field who recognize that many women would rather be treated by women, and who would like to see a specialist hospital set up for women, staffed by women.

In recent years, however, governments have been closing down our existing women's hospitals.

Women's reactions: anxious, afraid and confused

It takes two to be partners in health care. However, many women have strong inhibitions about their bodies. Just as doctors can get embarrassed about breasts, so can women patients – for the same cultural reasons.

Charlene Bargeron of the Breast Care Campaign believes that while most women are well-informed on other health issues, when it comes to breasts we have a blind spot:

> Women find it difficult to examine themselves, partly because of the sexual connotations of touching yourself, and partly because there is a belief that if you've got breast cancer you are going to die and some women don't want to know that. Many women are led to believe that their sexual attractiveness depends on their breasts, and that is all they have. Breasts are vital to their self-image and their sex life.

And ignorance about breasts – among women and health professionals alike – is alarmingly high. 'There are only two things we ever learn about breasts,' remarks Charlene, 'that they are an erogenous zone, and that they kill women through breast cancer. It's sex or death. Sex we don't talk about. As for death, we stick our heads in the sand.'

And what information is available for women about their breasts? Schools don't teach children about breast care. GPs' surgeries don't provide leaflets, and even the health professionals have trouble keeping up with developments in breast care. Not surprisingly, there is a crying need for information and reassurance when it comes to breasts.

When the Breast Care Campaign opened its telephone helpline in 1991, they were deluged with calls from women who were anxious, afraid and confused about their breasts. The helpline swiftly became a kind of anonymous confessional for up to thirty callers per session. Cancer was the greatest fear. (Nine out of ten women who find a breast lump believe it is malignant, yet in fact, nine out of ten breast lumps are harmless.)

A quarter of callers to the helpline hadn't been to a doctor. Some had lived for years with a secret fear, but felt unable to get help. Sometimes a friend or partner had telephoned for them, because the women would not even pick up the phone. A third of callers had seen their GP, but were still concerned about their breasts and said that their GP had not reassured them. Others said that their GP was unsympathetic or patronizing and had just told them 'not to worry'.

The majority of calls to the helpline were about breast pain, which affects most pre-menopausal women at some time. 'Women tend to put up with breast pain in a state of fear,' says Charlene Bargeron. 'They are told it is part and parcel of being a woman.' The next largest category of callers wanted to talk about breast lumps and discharge. (For remedies, see Chapter Nine.)

These are some examples of calls the helpline received:

- A father called on behalf of his fourteen-year-old daughter after her doctor suggested surgery for a breast lump (at this age any lump is almost certainly harmless).
- A woman had been offered a mastectomy for her breast pain (apart from the mutilation involved, this may not be an effective treatment).
- Other women were concerned about being put on HRT by their doctors without breast examinations or discussion of the cancer risks (see Chapter Ten).
- One woman was extremely unhappy with her breasts because her skin was transparent enough to reveal her veins.
- Others rang after seeing doctors about pain or nipple discharge and being told to 'put up with it, it's a woman's lot'.
- One woman was very upset after her GP had told her, 'I don't deal in breasts.'
- A woman in her seventies rang to say that many years ago she had been given a radical mastectomy for breast cancer. Today, in the knowledge that such drastic surgery does not improve chances of survival, she is still tormented by feelings of bitterness and rage.
- One woman went to see her GP about a lump. He wasn't worried. She was. He arranged for her to have a mammogram, but it didn't alleviate her anxiety because he didn't explain the meaning of 'mammogram'.

According to one of the helpline nurses:

Most women want to talk to someone about what the GP has said or not said. If they are very anxious, they can't take in what their

GP says anyway. When they get home they feel they can't talk to him [sic] again, in case he thinks they are silly, or wasting his time. It's easier to talk to a nurse, so they ring us and say, 'I'm sorry to bother you, but I've got this lump and I'm so worried, I haven't slept for a week.'

The campaign worked hard to get sponsorship to keep its helpline going. Charlene Bargeron tried bra manufacturers. Most were unhelpful: 'They had never thought about breast care from the health point of view before.' The helpline was closed in 1992, due to lack of funding.

'Put birdseed in your bra . . .'

For the minority of women (about one in ten) whose breast problem does turn out to be cancer, their emotional and psychological experience of the disease can be quite as bruising as the physical trauma. While researching this book, I spoke with staff and volunteers at Breast Cancer Care in London.

As the only breast cancer charity in this country which specializes in supporting women with breast cancer, Breast Cancer Care receives some 10,000 calls to its telephone helpline every year and supports many thousands more women. All Breast Cancer Care volunteers have themselves been through the experience of cancer and breast surgery.

The overriding impression they gave me was that many women with this disease feel a lot of anger and hurt about the way they are treated – as women, as patients, as 'breasts'. Just as women feel deep and lasting distress about bad experiences in hospital when they are giving birth, so women who have been to hospital for breast cancer have a fund of tales to tell, often involving astonishing insensitivity on the part of doctors.

In 1992, Breast Cancer Care was contacted regarding a recent mastectomy patient who had been given no information about a prosthesis or reconstruction. When she asked for help, this woman's surgeon had recommended sewing up a bag of birdseed to put in her bra. Breast Cancer Care sent two information packs: one for the woman, one for her doctor.

Another call to Breast Cancer Care came from a woman who – in the absence of advice about reconstruction or prosthesis – had been told by her doctor to 'roll up a pair of knickers and stuff them in your bra'.

Other calls are from women who feel they have met with apparent indifference and coldness when what they need most is information and support. Andrea Whalley, the former director of Breast Cancer Care, explains:

> I had a call from a woman who was very angry and she asked specifically to talk to me to be sure that Breast Cancer Care's director was aware of what was going on. She went into hospital at 9 a.m. Her surgery was in the afternoon. Nobody talked to her at all about what was going to happen. Within 48 hours of surgery she was sent home as she was – with a drain still in her chest – and no advice about how to deal with the consequences of her mastectomy. She was a widow living on her own and she was very angry, frightened and distraught.

One of Breast Cancer Care's staff adds:

> Nobody talked to me at all when I went in for my mastectomy. I sat there thinking – somebody will talk to me today. Nobody smiles at you either. You think, 'I'm going to die'. That was fourteen

years ago, but things have changed very little since then. That's
why breast care nurses [trained to discuss your treatment and your
feelings with you] are so important.

These bad experiences can't all be blamed on doctors. Breast
cancer itself is bound to cause a wealth of difficult feelings in any
woman, including anger and depression. And even when we are
healthy, many of us suffer from the sense that our breasts don't
really belong to us. In our culture, breasts are public property –
which generally means male property (see Chapters One and
Two).

The point is that when women go for breast-cancer treatment,
they carry these feelings with them and find they are com-
pounded: women often say they are expected to 'hand their bodies
over' to doctors, to step on to a 'conveyor belt' of medical care.

Some breast-cancer patients complain they have no sense of
control over their treatment (although some women do prefer to
rely on doctors and gladly give up the burden of responsibility).
Another problem for women is lack of information and lack of
choice in treatments. Often doctors can't give women the information they want because no one really knows the answers.

Should women start asking for information and choice, they
may be seen as 'difficult' or 'neurotic'. Many doctors seem to feel
threatened by women's questions, perhaps because it is hard for
them to deal with their own feelings about the pain and uncer-
tainty of this disease.

One Breast Cancer Care volunteer puts some of this defensive-
ness on the part of GPs down to the lack of consensus about
breast cancer, and the competitiveness of medics in finding
the right answers. 'Cancer is about a contest between clinicians
to show who is right in their treatment,' she says. 'It's an
adversarial system.'

It isn't easy for a doctor to admit that he or she has no clear answers, no 'cure' for breast cancer. It isn't easy for doctors to deal with 'failure', or a patient's grief and possible death.

So women may be faced with their doctor's difficulties, as well as their own shock and distress. 'It's very scary for doctors to have women wanting to know what is going on,' said one breast cancer counsellor. 'What you need at that point is emotional courage to face their negative response. But that is very difficult at the time.'

Time for change

The image of the breast itself, identified as it is in our society with sex and femininity, is hurtful to women who have had breast surgery.

'Women often say that all those cleavages – in advertisements and hoardings and on television – just "come out and hit you",' remarked one breast cancer counsellor. Clare Short, the MP who campaigned against 'topless' pictures in newspapers, has talked of the daily hurt felt by a woman with a mastectomy when her husband kept bringing home tabloids featuring the page-three 'lovelies'.

'The cultural razzmatazz about breasts,' says a Breast Cancer Care volunteer, also obscures the fact that 'our breasts are important to us, as people. They are not just sexual or maternal. They are intrinsic.'

Penny Brohn, who was at first branded a 'rebel' in medical circles when she refused conventional cancer treatments and founded the Bristol Cancer Help Centre, believes that cancer itself opens a Pandora's box of feelings – in everyone who comes into contact with it. In her book *Gentle Giants*, she writes:

> Cancer seems to evoke in the average man [sic] much the same emotions as it does in the people who have it. These include disgust, guilt, grief, and of course, that good old favourite, fear . . . Just when I needed a lot of support and affection I had to cope with projected fear and rejection, which was hard.

We need to challenge the stereotyped ideas about breasts and bring breast cancer into the light of day if we are to air those feelings and dispel that fear.

Thanks to the courage of many women who have survived breast cancer, that process has begun. Says one woman who had a mastectomy some years ago:

> I'd never met anyone with breast cancer at the time. Nobody talked about it. I didn't tell anyone about my own. That has changed now.

Professor Barry Gusterson of the Institute of Cancer Research and of Breakthrough, has also noticed a change:

> Twenty years ago nobody talked about the subject. Women with breast cancer kept it quiet. That is changing and people are much more open these days.

But we also need to change attitudes in the medical profession, because if women fear their complex feelings about their breasts are not going to be respected, then they will be slow to come forward for health care.

The penalty of this fear (intensified by the fear of cancer) could be death. Eight thousand women a year in the UK don't get treatment for breast cancer until a dangerously late stage. We will have to change attitudes to breasts – which means changing attitudes to women – before we get the sensitive and effective health care we need.

Women have already successfully campaigned to alter many social and medical attitudes to pregnancy and childbirth. The pressure is now on from women who want more choice, more information, more financial resources and more sensitivity in the treatment of breast diseases too.

9
The unwell breast

When health problems develop

Just as most of us know little about the workings of the well breast, we also know little about the common and relatively harmless disorders that bother half of all women from time to time.

This chapter is about the many benign (i.e. non-cancerous) breast disorders that make up nine-tenths of all breast health problems. They vary from the common symptoms of breast pain to less common nipple disorders and breast lumps. Some are uncomfortable, some can be very painful, but none of them is life-threatening.

Yet there is no need for women to suffer in silence – breast pain is real pain – and no need to put up with doctors who don't take these problems seriously. There are effective self-help remedies for many benign breast problems, as well as some effective drug treatments.

What is 'normal' and what is 'disease'?

Nine out of ten women who go to a breast clinic for health problems will be told that they have one of the common, non-cancerous disorders classed as 'benign breast disease'. But the word disease is misleading: many of the symptoms women have – like lumpiness, tenderness and swelling – are simply part of the wide range of changes women's breasts normally go through.

The latest thinking is that benign conditions are part of a spectrum which reaches from 'normal' through 'mild aberration' to 'disease'. The difficulty for doctors is in deciding where normality ends and disease begins.

Fortunately, many benign breast disorders have effective remedies, ranging from a change in diet to prescription drugs. Even when women don't have treatment, more than half of benign conditions will eventually go away of their own accord.

Battling with fear

When we have pain, infections or lumps in other parts of our bodies, most of us don't hesitate to do something about it. Whether it's tonsils or toes, backache or bellyache, we can tell friends, family or GP.

But when it comes to our breasts, what do we do? We assume 'the worst'! Many of us wait for months in anxious silence, hoping that the problem will just go away. If it's going to be a fatal disease, we rationalize, there's nothing we can do. If it's not going to be a fatal disease, there's no need to do anything.

Our fear is founded upon a widespread, national ignorance of benign breast problems. These make up the vast proportion of breast complaints, but they are not dramatic and most of us have never heard of them. They are mostly part of the spectrum of 'normal' breast changes women experience throughout their lives and they get little media coverage. In this country, too, benign breast disease is of little interest to the drug companies who nowadays fund much research, because there are few drugs to be sold in this field, few profits to be made.

And so benign breast problems attract few headlines, few research grants, no glory. In the words of cancer specialist Ian Fentiman (Guy's Hospital) writing in *Lancet* (vol. 335):

> There has always been a discrepancy between the workload of breast clinics and publications on the subject of breast diseases. Thus 90 per cent of symptomatic patients have benign conditions, whereas 95 per cent of publications concern aspects of breast cancer.

There are other, related reasons why women don't want to deal with or think about their breast problems, and these are to do with doctors and the way we think of breasts – and of women – in our culture (see Chapter Eight).

There can also be acute embarrassment at the very prospect of having our breasts examined by our GP, especially if he is male, especially if we live in small communities. What's more, many doctors don't take non-cancerous breast problems seriously. They assume that women with breast pain are 'neurotic' and they can be very patronizing and dismissive to their patients. Women who know this from personal experience or through the grapevine are reluctant to put themselves through the ordeal of a medical examination.

Armed with the facts, however, we can avoid the terrible anxiety which is often the worst symptom of a benign breast disorder. And we can find the best treatment, whether through self-help or through a sympathetic GP.

By any other name

Half of us will have some kind of benign breast disorder in the years between puberty and the menopause. You are more likely to suffer from one of these if other women in your family have had breast disorders, or if you have irregular periods.

Yet there is still great confusion about what to call the various breast disorders, and every country has its own classification. There are over a hundred terms for painful, lumpy breasts. In the 1930s for instance, the term 'chronic mastitis' was often used, mistakenly, for breast pain. And as late as 1923, the treatment for 'chronic mastitis' was mastectomy. Some doctors still (mistakenly) call breast pain 'mastitis'.

Fortunately, that has changed, but 'a lot of nonsensical notions have persisted,' says Professor Robert Mansel, a world authority on benign breast disease:

> Every day of the week, GPs still prescribe antibiotics for painful breasts, although this is totally illogical. Painful breasts are a hormonal condition: you wouldn't get a GP prescribing antibiotics for other hormonal conditions like thyroid problems.

Names are important when it comes to telling women what they are suffering from. Being told you have a 'disease' is frightening, needlessly so when much pain and lumpiness is 'normal' and when breast pain has no link with cancer. Most women with painful, lumpy breasts have no greater risk of breast cancer than any other woman.

Why is there such confusion in pinning down breast disorders? Because the breast itself is very complex, and so is the life cycle of a woman. The breast changes enormously – and not in any orderly way – throughout our lives. According to Professor Mansel:

Some parts of the breast are growing and others are regressing at the same time. For instance, what is sometimes called 'cystic disease' is actually a normal process of ageing in breast tissue.

The 'inverted iceberg'

In fact 'benign breast disease' is not really a disease at all. Rather it is a process of change. To try to make sense of this jumble, Mansel and his colleagues came up with the 'ANDI' (Aberrations of Normal Development and Involution) classification technique. ANDI provides a way of placing breast changes – which are mostly normal – on a spectrum of change (for instance: 'normal', 'aberration', 'disease').

To give an idea of how comparatively harmless most breast changes are, Professor Mansel uses the metaphor of the 'inverted iceberg'. The most common and noticeable (usually meaning painful) complaints which women take to their GPs are the least dangerous. Yet, invisible below the water-line, and therefore often unnoticed, are the small minority of complaints which signal serious disease.

A modern problem

Modern industrial societies have brought rapid and dramatic changes to women's bodies. Our reproductive patterns have altered out of all recognition in a very short period of time and, although we are under strong cultural pressure to ignore the fact, our breasts are an integral part of our reproductive systems.

Our ancestors may have had only half a dozen periods in their entire lifetimes. Much of the time they would have been pregnant, or breastfeeding fully (which halts ovulation and menstruation), and many of them died long before the age when breast disease becomes a worry for modern women.

In contrast, today's Western woman starts her periods earlier than ever (from about twelve), and doesn't reach the menopause until she is in her fifties. The only breaks in the menstrual cycle come when she has a child or two (she may not have any), and when she breastfeeds (she may not breastfeed for long, or at all). As a result, she may have three or four hundred periods in her life. And with each period, hormones surge through her body, her breasts change – and change back again. Under the circumstances it's not surprising that things go wrong from time to time.

Breast pain

Of all breast conditions, pain is the one that women seek help for most often. This kind of pain is not necessarily confined to the breast. It may be felt at the top inner part of the arm. Often it is the fear of cancer which is as big a problem as the pain itself.

Breast pain, also known as mastalgia, varies in intensity from minor discomfort to long-term, disabling agony. Because there have been few studies into mastalgia, we know little about it, and little about how to treat it. But broadly speaking, there are two types of breast pain.

Cyclical pain is the most common type of breast pain. It is worst before a period, and it tends to affect women in their late twenties and thirties. Non-cyclical pain is more common in women over forty, and it can occur at any time. There are good treatments (see below) for both types of pain, although premenstrual pain tends to be easier to treat.

1. Cyclical pain

Most of us know what it is like to have breasts which become tender, lumpy and/or swollen in the days before a period. The breasts may ache, or suffer from sharp shooting pains. But if you have pain in both breasts and it seems related to the timing of your periods, there is almost certainly nothing to worry about.

What happens is that our breasts prepare for pregnancy during each menstrual cycle by building up a lining designed to make milk. As our bodies realize that we are not pregnant, the tissue and fluid that make up this lining drain away. In most women, the lumpiness disappears too – until the next month.

One theory is that the problem stems from an abnormal sensitivity of breast tissue to our hormones. Diet can affect our sensitivity (see below), especially our consumption of fatty acids. Women with breast pain have low levels of GLA (gamolenic acid) and high levels of saturated fatty acids which appear to increase the effects of hormones on the breast, causing pain.

For many women with breast pain the relief of being told they haven't got cancer is all the treatment they want. The Cardiff Breast Clinic has found that the vast majority of women (85 per cent) were successfully treated by simple reassurance and a proper explanation of the nature of mastalgia.

There are other causes of cyclical breast pain. It may be a side-effect of HRT, the Pill or progestagen-only pills. Changing or stopping these treatments should end the pain.

But for some women breast pain can be longer lasting and far more severe, affecting the quality of a woman's life. Some women can't sleep at night for the pain, can't hug their children, can't bear to be touched. If you have this kind of pain, do ask to see a breast specialist and see below for treatments.

2. Non-cyclical pain

Some kinds of breast pain (one-third of cases) have no monthly pattern. This is called non-cyclical breast pain, and again, we know little about it. The pain may be in one breast, and it may be related to an accident, sports strain, injury or an infection. Breast pain is not uncommon in arthritic conditions of the ribs or of the neck. Sometimes an infection of the oesophagus (the gullet), or even heart problems, can cause referred pain in the breast.

For some girls painful breasts and nipples are a side-effect of growing up. If you have this problem, first get your breasts checked out by a doctor to rule out any other reasons. Then invest in a well-fitting bra to avoid friction with nipples. Painkillers like aspirin may also help.

But non-cyclical pain in one breast can occasionally, but rarely, turn out to be cancer. This kind of pain is usually localized and persistent. It's wise not to take chances with it. Do see your doctor.

Seeking help for breast pain

It is important not to ignore breast pain. Why should you put up with it? It is as 'real' as any other pain and is *not* in your mind.

Finding a doctor who will treat it sympathetically, however, is not always easy. You can ask to see another doctor. You may want to 'go shopping' for treatment, asking other women, making your own enquiries through organizations like those listed in the Appendix at the back of this book.

You may want to see a woman GP (there's a 50 per cent chance that she will have had breast pain herself), although not all women GPs are as sympathetic as women would like.

Ideally, your treatment for breast pain should start when your sympathetic doctor checks that you don't have cancer and gives you full reassurance of that fact. You may also want to keep a breast pain chart to establish whether your pain is *cyclical* or *non-cyclical* – and which would be the best treatments.

After that, you may want to try some of the self-help measures suggested below.

Self-help   Many women say that the following measures have helped them to beat breast pain without having to undergo drug treatments.

- Cut down on saturated fat in your diet (like those in meat and dairy foods).
- Try evening primrose oil. This is a remedy which has virtually no side-effects (2 per cent of women complain of flatulence or mild stomach upsets). However, you do need to take evening primrose oil for three or four months, taking four to six capsules a day, before it takes effect. It is also quite expensive to buy, and you will face quite an array of brands at your chemist or health shop. Preferably, ask your GP to prescribe it so that you get gamolenic acid (the active ingredient) in the right dosage. (Avoid using evening primrose oil, as you would avoid taking any medication during the first

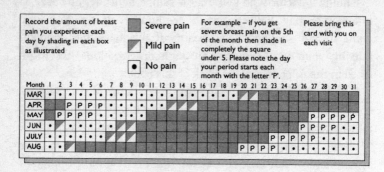

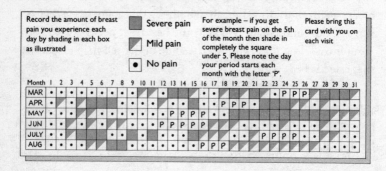

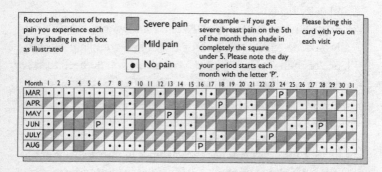

three months of pregnancy when the foetus is most vulnerable to abnormality.)

- Choose the right bra for you, so that you get both support and comfort. Bras that push your breasts upwards with underwiring or rigid frames can also dig into you, making you ache. Once you find a good bra (easier said than done), try wearing it at night as well as in the daytime if it helps.
- Cutting down on sugar can help, as can eating more fruit and vegetables.
- Losing weight can also mean more comfortable breasts as they grow smaller and lighter.
- Studies from the US also suggest that cutting down on caffeine can reduce breast pain. But American women tend to drink far more coffee and cola drinks than British women, and there is no evidence in this country that caffeine contributes to breast pain. On the other hand, there is no harm in trying it: your general health is likely to improve, at least.
- Stress may also be a factor in breast pain: it is known to have an effect on our hormones. Proven or not, it can't hurt any woman to try to reduce the stress in her life. Try relaxation techniques, or regular exercise, or meditation: they all help combat stress.
- Try to improve your posture. If you grew up with large breasts, you may be in the habit of rounding your shoulders

Figure 5: (a) Pain chart of a patient with cyclical pronounced mastalgia showing 2–3 weeks of severe to mild mastalgia per cycle over 6 months. (b) Pain chart showing a non-cyclical pattern of mastalgia. (c) Pain chart of a patient who subsequently developed a small palpable cancer at the site of pain. Source: Hughes, L.E., Mansel, R.E. and Webster, D., *Benign Disorders and Diseases of the Breast*, Baillière Tindall, 1989

to disguise them. Or you may spend the day working over a desk. Good posture and breathing exercises can counteract the hunching tendency. A yoga class may help with both. The Alexander Technique is also good for posture.

- Some complementary therapists advise 'water therapy' for a range of benign breast problems, especially tenderness and swelling. Spray your breasts with cold water once or twice a day to promote circulation and 'tone-up' the breast tissue.
- Breast exercises can also help, and can be combined with water therapy. Cath Cirket in her book *Breast Health* recommends three types of simple exercise:

    1. Press the palms of your hands together in front of your breasts.
    2. Grip your hands together in front of your breasts, and pull your fingers away from each other.
    3. Grasp your forearms in front of your breasts, pulling your arms away from each other.

Medical help   However reassurance and self-help remedies are not always enough. There are women who suffer such severe breast pain that they are desperate for a solution. According to Professor Mansel:

> Women have come to my clinic in floods of tears. They say, 'I've been all over the country looking for help and no doctor will listen to me; they all say I'm crazy.' Some plead with me to give them mastectomies to put them out of their pain. I may spend up to two hours talking with them. What they want as much as anything is an admission that there are some things we doctors don't understand.

In fact, surgery has little place in the treatment of breast pain. Mastectomy doesn't work; even after the breast has gone, pain can persist, rather as it does in a phantom limb. Fortunately, the

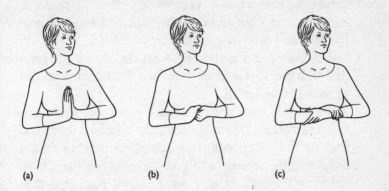

(a)   (b)   (c)

Figure 6: Three simple exercises
1 Press the palms of your hands together in front of your breasts.
2 Gripping your hands together in front of your breasts, pull your fingers away from each other.
3 Grasping your forearms in front of your breasts, pull your arms away from each other.
Source: Cirket, C., *A Woman's Guide to Breast Health*, Thorsons, 1992

drug treatments are effective in treating most women, especially for cyclical breast pain. In half of women, the pain does recur, but often in a milder form. As with the problems of menstrual pain, we don't fully understand the mechanics of breast pain.

There are various medical treatments which have had some success in treating severe breast pain:

• Efamast – gamolenic acid (GLA), the active ingredient in evening primrose oil, can now be prescribed by your doctor. Unfortunately, some GPs are reluctant to prescribe efamast because of costs. Efamast is available over the counter. However, get a prescription from your doctor if you can. This will ensure that you get GLA in the right dosage. You should also have a breast examination to check for cancer at the same time. (Efamast is only licensed for use as a drug in the treatment of breast pain, and not for PMT.)

- The combined oral contraceptive pill can also help a great deal with breast pain in some women, but not all of us can or want to take the Pill.
- There are two other drugs for breast pain called bromocriptine and danazol. These are powerful hormonal drugs and they do have some disturbing side-effects in more than a quarter of the women who take them. Danazol is a male hormone that can literally put hairs on your chin (hirsutism). It also interferes with women's periods (amenorrhoea), can cause oily skin, weight gain, muscle aches and voice changes (sometimes permanent). Bromocriptine causes nausea and dizziness in a third of women who take it. You must also use barrier contraceptives if you take these drugs.

Breast lumps

It's what so many of us have learned to dread: finding a lump in our breasts. But only one in twelve breast lumps is cancerous and the rest are usually harmless. Cancer is also rare in younger people, but it becomes more prevalent later in life.

If you are familiar with your breasts you will know that normal breast tissue is more or less lumpy anyway, depending on the stage of your menstrual cycle.

The kind of lumps you are looking for when you examine yourself (see p. 131) are quite distinct from the normal, lumpy tissue. They are big: probably about an inch across, or the size of

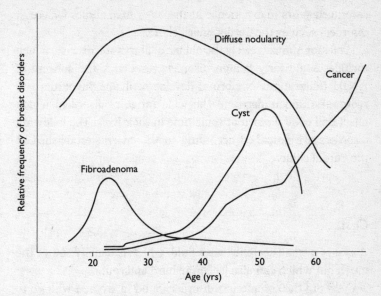

Figure 7: Age distribution of breast disorders. Source: I C R F Factsheet 6.10

a grape. They feel different. They stick out. (This applies to cancerous lumps too: you won't be able to feel a malignant lump when it is small.)

There are various types of breast lumps. One type is cancerous. The others are all benign, but they have many different names.

You may have heard of so-called fibrocystic disease which covers *any* non-cancerous growth in the breast. But this book doesn't use this term. As we have seen, there is still tremendous confusion amongst doctors about what to call breast disorders – as well as how to treat them. This book follows the terminology and classifications of Professor Robert Mansel and his colleagues, whose book *Benign Disorders and Diseases of the Breast* is based on seventeen years of experience at the specialized clinics for breast disorders such as the Cardiff breast clinic.

Professor Mansel rejects the old term 'fibrocystic disease' which includes some forty benign disorders, and uses the concept of ANDI (aberrations of normal development and involution) to reorganize and understand the wide range of disorders which affect half of all women at some time in their lives. The following disorders are described according to the criteria established at the Cardiff clinic.

Cysts

A cyst is a small sac filled with fluid, which is usually soft to the touch but which can also feel quite hard and round.

Cysts are the commonest disorder found in women who go to a breast clinic. Up to seven per cent of us will have a breast cyst at some time during our reproductive lives. They can grow in one or both breasts as a result of a change (aberration) in the normal process of ageing (involution) of the breast's lobules.

Cysts can grow quite big, and they can also cluster together to seem like one large lump. They can feel painful and tender, but they are benign. They are common in women approaching the menopause, but can occur from your thirties onwards. Most studies show no connection between cysts and cancer.

Their medical treatment is simple, relatively painless, and can be done on the spot in a hospital breast clinic. According to Professor Mansel *et al:*

> The first investigation of every lump in the breast should be the insertion of a needle, and if this is practised, cysts will be diagnosed at first consultation. A 21-gauge needle with a syringe of appropri-

ate size to the estimated cyst volume is plunged directly into the cyst, fixed by two fingers of the (doctor's) opposite hand. No anaesthetic is necessary. Once all the fluid has been removed, the needle comes out and the fluid is thrown away. Then the breast should be carefully felt to make sure there is no other lump. If there is, it should be re-needled to draw out tissue for further examination.

Professor Mansel lays down two cardinal rules for doctors in the safe aspiration (removal with a needle) of cysts:

1. The mass must disappear completely after aspiration. If not, it should be examined again using techniques such as mammography, ultrasound and biopsy with a needle to obtain cells for a diagnosis.
2. The fluid must not be bloodstained. If it is, the doctor should take a biopsy to examine the lump further.

If the lump turns out to be solid, a specimen is taken by aspirating cells with the needle and this is passed on to the laboratory for further testing.

Some women get cysts over and over again, sometimes in the same place, sometimes in a new part of the breast. Recurrent cysts can be aspirated many times, but they rarely refill after two or three aspirations. The treatment has an immediate effect, rather like collapsing a balloon. It may leave the breast a little sore or bruised.

There are various confusing and alarming names – like fibroadenosis, or chronic cystic mastitis, or fibrocystic disease, or cystic breast disease – sometimes used to describe the condition which produces cysts.

There is also another uncommon type of cyst called the 'galactocele'. This shows up as a painless swelling of the breast some weeks or even months after a woman has stopped breast-feeding. The swelling has exactly the same characteristics as the usual breast cyst except that the fluid it contains is milk, as opposed to the usual cyst fluids. Cysts are usually found near the areola.

Fibroadenomas

A fibroadenoma is a benign growth of fibrous and glandular tissue. Fibroadenosis is another general term used to describe painful, lumpy areas in the breast.

In contrast to cysts, fibroadenomas are lumps that commonly crop up in young women and teenagers. But like cysts, they are common, harmless (except in the anxiety they may cause you) and have no links with cancer.

Fibroadenomas feel smooth and rubbery, and they move around easily in the breast tissue. They are usually marble-sized, or they may be as big as a lemon. They are usually noticed accidentally by young women when they are bathing or getting dressed.

A doctor may want to check that your lump is not a cancer by performing a needle aspiration to take out some cells. But fibroadenomas don't always have to be removed. Some doctors suggest just leaving them alone in younger women. But in older women it may be wiser to remove them to make sure they are not cancerous. The procedure may take fifteen minutes in an operating theatre under general anaesthetic, followed by a night or two in hospital. A district nurse may later remove the stitches, or they may dissolve. However, these lumps are increasingly being removed under local anaesthetic, without requiring a stay in hospital.

A lactational fibroadenoma is one which develops during pregnancy.

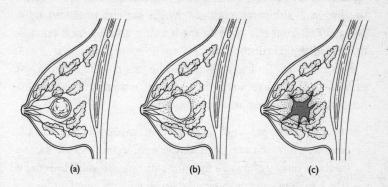

Figure 8: This diagram shows the mobility of breast lumps in relation to the surrounding breast tissue. The shaded area shows the amount of breast tissue which 'moves' with the lump. (a) Fibroadenoma (b) Cyst (c) Cancer. Source: Hughes, L.E., Mansel, R.E. and Webster, D., *Benign Disorders and Diseases of the Breast*, Baillière Tindall, 1989

Fat necrosis

Very rarely, lumps in the breast occur after a severe blow has caused the death of fat cells. This is not a serious condition, but it is important to know about fat necrosis because the lumps it produces feel just like cancers.

We all experience the occasional knock on the breast which can do no long-term harm. But a severe blow to the breast can be enough to burst open fat cells. The body reacts to the fat by bundling it up in scar tissue, making a firm, irregular lump. When the scar tissue contracts, it pulls on the breast's suspensory ligaments, producing skin dimpling and a change in the shape of the breast – the same changes which can be produced by a cancer. This kind of a blow to the breast is usually hard enough to cause definite bruising.

According to Professor Mansel, the main danger from fat necrosis is that doctors will miss cancer, assuming that a breast lump has been caused by a blow instead:

> In spite of the universal teaching that fat necrosis can simulate cancer, procrastination with cancer still occurs because doctors accept a history of trauma from the patient . . . It would be better if the condition were unknown, for it is sufficiently rare that no one would be disadvantaged if it were unrecognized. Breast cancer is [estimated to be] forty times more common. We would put the figures even higher.

There are two types of fat necrosis. The first kind occurs in mostly older women and it resembles cancer. The second kind occurs in younger women – for instance women in their forties who might have had a car accident – and it resembles a cyst.

The first kind, to be diagnosed safely, means you must have a needle biopsy. Mammography and cytology (examination of the cells under a microscope) may also be helpful. Usually, the lump will be removed surgically under general anaesthetic, involving a short stay in hospital.

The second kind can be diagnosed using mammography, and it can be removed using aspiration (the fluid is withdrawn using a needle attached to a syringe). This procedure can be done on the spot at a breast clinic, without anaesthetic. However fat necrosis usually means a solid lump which can't be treated by aspiration.

Sclerosing adenosis

This is a benign breast condition caused by new glandular growth in the breast which has become hardened (sclerosing means hardening). The result is that the breasts produce easily felt lumps or lumpiness. The breasts can also feel painful and tender. If a duct under the nipple is affected, the nipple may turn inwards. It is also considered one of the manifestations of ANDI (see p. 168) – in other words it is one of the benign disorders which comes with ageing.

Sclerosing adenosis is mostly a condition which occurs in women in their forties and fifties. It is treated as any other breast lump, by assessments at a breast clinic including mammography and the study of cells (cytology) after biopsy. If a cancer cannot be ruled out at this stage, the lump may be surgically removed, under general anaesthetic, possibly involving a short stay in hospital.

Nipple problems

It can be alarming to find that your nipples are producing liquid when you don't expect it. But usually it is nothing to worry about. Most nipple discharge is due to simple, benign causes.

Most women do have some amount of discharge when their nipples are squeezed, whether they are pregnant, not pregnant, old or young. Even newborn babies can have some wetness from their nipples (called 'witches' milk'), a result of the hormones in their mothers' blood. This is all quite normal.

During pregnancy, many women find that their nipples leak

drops of milk, too. Even many years after you have finished with breastfeeding you may be able to express a little milk from your nipples. (But treat them gently and never squeeze them on a regular basis.)

Sometimes, an excess of the hormone prolactin can make a woman who has never been pregnant appear to produce milk. Taking the Pill can have this effect, as can other drugs.

You should only be concerned about nipple discharge when it happens on one side but not the other, and when it comes out by itself over a period of time. This liquid may be clear and sticky, or it may be bloody. See your doctor about it. It could be caused by a benign wart-like growth on the duct called a duct papilloma, or it could be a collection of these little warts called intraductal papillomatosis.

Alternatively it may be caused by a 'pre-cancer' which clogs the duct (intraductal carcinoma *in situ*), or in rare cases it may be cancer. Less than 4 per cent of women with a nipple discharge have cancer.

If you find a nipple discharge on your clothes, the wisest course of action is to see your doctor.

Duct ectasia

Duct ectasia is the enlarging and eventually the hardening of a diseased duct accompanied by discharge from the nipple. It can happen in one or both breasts. Usually, it is women in their forties who are affected. This is not a common condition, but it can be a cause of three common breast symptoms: lumps, nipple discharge and pain – as well as nipple inversion.

Duct ectasia occurs when a duct fills with cellular waste products making a sticky discharge which can vary in colour from cream to green to bloody. The discharge may be as thick as toothpaste. Sometimes there will be a burning or itching feeling in the nipples, too. In time, the diseased ducts harden, pulling the nipple inwards. There will be a hard lumpiness in the nipple area. The surrounding skin may become dimpled or red, and there may be swelling in the lymph nodes under the arms.

Not much is known about the causes of this disorder, and in extreme cases doctors are unsure about the best treatments. Simple duct ectasia with a small degree of nipple discharge may clear up without medical treatment. But in more difficult cases – and these may include severe infections – doctors may try various drugs such as antibiotics, together with surgical drainage. Occasionally, doctors will want to operate to remove the affected ducts. However, women can't breastfeed after such operations, and they can also lose sensation in their nipples.

Duct papillomas

A papilloma is a small, benign, wart-like growth. A duct papilloma (or intraductal papilloma) is one that grows in the milk duct beneath the nipple. Some are too small to feel: others are as big as a pea. They usually show up first with drops of blood from the nipple – coming from the same duct of the nipple each time. This is a common condition during the years of monthly, cyclical change and there is little, if any, risk of it causing cancer.

A common symptom is nipple discharge which varies in colour from bloody to green. Sometimes an intraductal papilloma can cause the nipple to turn inwards or it can cause dimpling in the skin of the breast. Usually, this is not a painful condition. Occasionally, there is inflammation or change in the shape or size of the breast, and the nipple may become inverted. Treatment

176 The unwell breast

usually involves cutting out the papilloma, a minor operation performed under a general anaesthetic. A cut is made down the side of the nipple and the offending duct is removed. If there is any doubt about which duct is involved, all the ducts will be cut out, using an incision around the lower edge of the areola.

Itching and soreness

Some girls and women suffer from itchy nipples. This can be irritating, but it is rarely serious. Young women may find their skin becomes itchy as their breasts grow. Others will have itchiness from dry skin, or an allergic reaction to their bra or detergent. (A soothing lotion like calamine can help.) Some women also suffer from eczema on their nipples.

One condition which can be confused with an eczema-type rash is in fact a kind of cancer called Paget's disease. So if you have a rash that doesn't respond to standard treatments, ask your doctor's opinion.

Sore nipples have a number of causes. They can be – in men and women – a result of jogging. 'Jogger's nipple' happens when the nipples rub against clothes during running. The nipples may become so chafed that they will bleed. The solutions include wearing a firmer bra, and placing sticking tape over the nipples while jogging.

Sore nipples are also a common problem for women who are breastfeeding. Soreness and cracks in the nipple can make feeding very painful. Sore nipples are often caused by babies not being positioned properly on the breast. They may also be caused by thrush on the skin, for which your doctor can prescribe a cream, plus drops for the baby.

Dermatitis and eczema of the nipples can also cause soreness: creams are available for these conditions, from your doctor or chemist.

Breast infections

Breast infections can occur as localized problems, or as part of an illness of the whole body such as tuberculosis or syphilis. However, these diseases are now quite rare in this country.

The more common infections are easy to spot, but the rarer ones may be confusingly like cancer. Breast infections never lead to breast cancer, but some breast cancers do lead to infections, or can look like infections.

If you do get an infection, make an appointment to see your doctor. It can't cause cancer, and it can be treated.

Mastitis

Mastitis is the most common kind of breast infection. It usually occurs when women are breastfeeding (lactational mastitis): a milk duct may get blocked up with thick milk that doesn't flow very well. Milk is the ideal medium for encouraging the growth of bacteria, and bacteria can easily enter the breast from the baby's mouth through cracks in the nipple.

The result is a rapid infection causing a reddened, hot and painful breast. You may experience a high fever and achy, flu-like symptoms as well.

There are a number of steps you can take in the early stages of mastitis. Keep on suckling your baby as often as possible: this will help to draw out the milk and keep the duct clear. (The bacteria won't hurt the child: it will be destroyed by the baby's stomach acids.)

Some women also use hot compresses or baths, together with massage, to unblock the duct. Unfortunately, the heat may have the effect of speeding the bacterial growth. Other women try cold compresses or ice packs. These slow the growth of bacteria, but may also harden the milk.

The next step is usually antibiotics, which usually work very quickly. However, antibiotics can cause some unpleasant side-effects such as thrush, and many complementary therapists will say that antibiotics treat only the symptoms of the illness while undermining the body's own capacity to heal itself. (If you do take antibiotics, eating live yoghurt and/or taking lactobacillus tablets will help redress some of the side-effects.)

In about one in ten cases of mastitis, antibiotics don't work. Instead, the mastitis develops into an abscess, which has to be drained by a doctor. This can be done with a needle under local anaesthetic, but bigger abscesses may need a small operation under general anaesthetic. The wound is left open with a drain inserted, and the patient must stay in hospital for three or four days until the drain can come out. They may also be given intravenous antibiotics.

There should be no need to stop breastfeeding after treatment for an abscess.

In her *Book of Breastfeeding*, published by the National Childbirth Trust, Mary Smale suggests that feeding the baby with your breast hanging down (by putting the baby on the floor or a low table) can help mastitis. She also makes these recommendations to breastfeeding women who find that mastitis is a recurring problem:

- Check the baby's positioning in case one part of the breast is being neglected.
- Make sure your fingers are not pressing into the breast tissue as you feed.
- Cut down on animal fats.
- Cut down on tea, coffee and cola drinks, as well as any cigarettes.
- Eat well.
- Ask your doctor to take a culture of milk to see if a more appropriate antibiotic might be necessary – or a longer course.
- Ask for a swab of the baby's nose and throat in case he/she keeps giving you an infection.

Women tend to have high hopes of the satisfaction and fulfilment that can come with breastfeeding, so when things go wrong, you can feel very low. Try the National Childbirth Trust for help and advice about this.

Sometimes, women who are not breastfeeding develop mastitis (non-lactational mastitis). Treatment is usually with antibiotics such as penicillin. Abscesses can also occur in women who are not breastfeeding. Both these conditions, although rare, can mask cancer so it is important to have them checked by a doctor.

The second most common type of infection – although rare – is an abscess in the nipple (sub-areolar abscess). This happens when the secretions in the sebaceous glands get infected, causing a red, hot and sore area on the border of the nipple which looks like a boil. It looks and feels very nasty, but it will not be cancerous.

If this infection is caught at a very early stage it can be cured with antibiotics. If not, it may need to be opened and drained, either under a local or a general anaesthetic. Unfortunately, this infection tends to recur, and some doctors will eventually remove the gland by surgery. Even then, the problem may crop up again. In some cases, the nipple can be removed altogether.

Male problems

The male breast develops in the same way as the female breast up until puberty, and men can also suffer from benign breast problems as well as from breast cancer.

Gynaecomastia is a condition which causes swelling of the male breast. It is usually caused by minor hormonal imbalance or by drugs, and is not serious. However it can be very embarrassing and upsetting, especially for younger men. Older men will need to be checked to make sure their swelling is not a cancer.

Treatment may be simply a matter of reassurance that this is not a serious problem. But drug treatments and surgical removal of the breast tissues are also an option.

Best breast care

In summary, there are many minor, and few distressing, disorders that can crop up in a woman's breasts in the course of her life.

Much of the time, what women want is sympathetic advice and reassurance that they do not have cancer. Don't ever feel that you will be 'wasting your doctor's time' in asking for an appointment about a breast problem. If it doesn't turn out to be serious, your doctor should be as pleased as you are. If it does turn out to be serious, having sought treatment quickly will certainly have helped.

Armed with greater knowledge about our own bodies, we can overcome fear – often the greatest enemy – and either treat ourselves or find the best help from an understanding doctor. In the 1990s it should no longer be necessary for women to put up with dismissive attitudes of doctors who see benign breast problems as a matter of 'neurosis'. If *your* doctor won't or can't treat your benign breast problem, you have a right to look for one who can.

10
Breast cancer: facing the fears

Taking the ostrich position

Breast cancer is not a cheery subject. Some of us can't bear to think about it, let alone talk about it:

> My mother won't discuss it or do anything about it. The shutters come down straight away. I tried to get her to go for breast screening, but she won't even talk about it.

> No, I never examine my breasts. It terrifies me. I'm quite convinced I'll get breast cancer one day.

This is a fear with more than one layer. Most apparent is the fear of losing a breast, which to some women spells a loss of femininity, attractiveness and sense of 'self'. But underlying that fear is a deeper fear of death which – in women who have the disease – tends to put other fears into the shade.

So deep are our anxieties that workers at Breast Cancer Care say that women tend to shy away from their literature on display at exhibitions, despite its clear and sympathetic presentation.

But if we let it take hold, fear adds to the danger of breast cancer. Fear stops us from going to a doctor quickly. Fear stops us finding out about this disease – what causes it, what options we have in treatment, how we can fight it. Fear keeps us

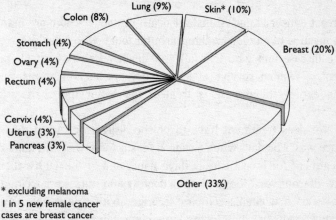

All neoplasms 124,000 (100%)

Lung (9%) Skin* (10%)
Colon (8%)
Stomach (4%) Breast (20%)
Ovary (4%)
Rectum (4%)
Cervix (4%)
Uterus (3%)
Pancreas (3%)
Other (33%)

* excluding melanoma
1 in 5 new female cancer
cases are breast cancer

Figure 9: The incidence of breast cancer in the UK. Source: Cancer Research Campaign Factsheet, 1988

ignorant, and ignorance makes us helpless.

And what we need when it comes to breast cancer is not helplessness but action. The level of breast cancer in this country is unnecessarily high. There is also a dearth of specialist care for women with breast cancer. All of us should be asking, 'Why does it still go on?' 'Why isn't more being done to save women's lives?'

Not a death sentence

Breast cancer is not an instant death sentence. There are many thousands of women walking around today who have survived the disease and who live full and healthy lives. About 60 per cent of women survive at least five years after diagnosis, and the earlier the disease is treated, the better the chances of recovery.

Nor does treatment have to be the disfiguring ordeal that it once was. The days when a radical mastectomy was the standard treatment for breast cancer have gone, and in the 1990s there are alternatives. More and more doctors and nurses are trying to respond to women's complex feelings about this disease. And complementary practitioners have made significant headway in their arguments for 'gentler' treatments that take the whole of a woman (mind, body and spirit) into account.

Since 1988 we have also had a nationwide screening programme which offers routine mammograms to women between the ages of fifty and sixty-four. Mammography can pick up signs of cancer in its earlier stages, and about 80 per cent of cancers found this way have a good prognosis.

Britain: highest death rate in the world for breast cancer

Yet one in twelve British women develops breast cancer at some time in her life. Fifteen thousand women a year die from it. There are 25,000 new cases a year. For women between the

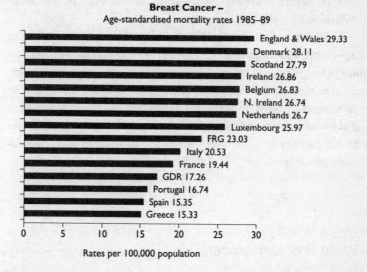

Figure 10: Breast cancer in the European Community. Source: Cancer Research Campaign Factsheet, 1992

ages of thirty-five and fifty-four, breast cancer is the most common single cause of death.

According to the statistics, this country has the worst death rate from breast cancer in the world, and this rate has not improved for thirty years.

There is no doubt that breast cancer is a very nasty and serious disease, not least because women who have been 'successfully' treated have to live with the knowledge that their cancer may come back again. The figures we have for past decades show that only one in five women had no further symptoms of the disease after treatment. (However, with the advent of the National Screening Programme which enables detection of tumours less than 2cms, these figures are set to improve dramatically as women with smaller tumours have less risk of symptoms recurring.)

And all too often, women's experience of breast cancer care in this country is disappointing. Women often complain that doctors are patronizing and insensitive, and those who want more information and choice may find themselves labelled 'neurotic' or 'hysterical'. Access to specialist team care in the UK – which should be every woman's right – is also very patchy. And many breast cancers (a third every year) are discovered at a dangerously late stage.

What is breast cancer?

The latest thinking is that breast cancer is a diverse and chronic disease of the whole body. There is no single type of breast cancer, and no single cure.

A cancer occurs when there is an uncontrolled reproduction of cells in the body. It may show up as a growth or a swelling. Not all growths are cancerous. There are also 'benign' growths which divide quickly, but these do not invade surrounding tissues or spread to other parts of the body.

Cancerous or 'malignant' growths do, however, invade other tissues and spread through the body. This happens when 'rogue' cancer cells break away from the original tumour and settle elsewhere to form 'secondaries'. This spread is called 'metastasis'. Cancer cells also lose their original function, becoming useless to the body, and they act as greedy parasites on other healthy tissues.

Breast cancer starts in the breast, but it spreads through the body from its earliest stages. According to Dr Susan Love, most breast cancers have been present for about nine years before you can even see them on a mammogram, and ten years before they can be felt as a lump. This means that cancers have had many years to spread microscopically through the lymph and blood systems before we can even detect them.

By the time a lump is big enough to feel, potential secondary tumours are already in place – although these may not develop for years to come. Of the 300 women who die of breast cancer every week, 60 per cent are killed by a secondary cancer.

Radical mastectomy then, is no longer seen as the 'cure' for breast cancer. The new, breast-conserving operation of lumpectomy – the removal of a section of the breast – may be just as effective in treating the tumour. But the whole body must be treated systemically to stop any secondary tumours from developing (see Chapter Eleven).

Yet mastectomies are still carried out. Why? Because sometimes a large area of the breast is affected. Or there may be a large tumour in a small breast. And sometimes women ask to have mastectomies, because they don't want to face the prospect of the cancer recurring in that breast.

It now seems that a woman's survival is determined not by surgery, but by the kind of tumour she has and by how well her immune system handles whatever cells have already spread from the breast.

What causes breast cancer?

Ask any two scientists what causes breast cancer and you are likely to get at least two answers, if not a healthy argument between them.

The factors involved in breast cancer – which itself comes in many forms and behaves differently in different women – are highly complex and interlinked. They are affected by culture, race, geography, lifestyle, diet, family and environmental factors.

Western women from industrialized nations have the highest breast cancer rate; women from the less 'developed' countries have the least. Sweden and the US have more breast cancer than we do in the UK, but statistically fewer deaths.

Japan has one of the lowest death rates from breast cancer in the world. Yet studies have shown that Japanese women who move to the US soon catch up with American breast cancer rates. For a long time, it was thought that a high intake of saturated animal fat in the diet might explain these differences. But other factors in the Western lifestyle, such as our patterns of childbearing, could be just as important.

What are your chances?

In any discussion of the risks of breast cancer it helps to remember three things:

Firstly, no one is certain what causes breast cancer, and the latest information can change very quickly.

Secondly, three-quarters of breast cancers occur in women with no known risk factors.

And thirdly, there is a human tendency to blame the victim – especially for frightening diseases that have sexual implications (witness the attitudes to people with AIDS). It may be true that breast cancer is linked to being overweight, or to having few babies later in life. That does not mean getting breast cancer is 'our fault', as if we could have prevented it by going on a diet (being more 'disciplined') or giving up a career for children (being less 'selfish').

If blame is to be laid, it is on our whole culture, not on individual women who live according to the expectations of that culture. And in any case, many women would choose to put up with the risks of Western living, rather than have children at an early age or change our diet just to minimize the risk of getting cancer. Many of the risk factors, too – like 'being tall' or having a relative with breast cancer – are beyond our control.

There is also a common belief that your personality has something to do with developing cancer. Some studies have suggested that women who 'bottle up' their feelings are at greater risk, and that 'determined' women will recover better from cancer.

'There is not a shred of evidence for the "cancer personality" view,' says Judy Deacon, a breast cancer epidemiologist at the Institute for Cancer Research. 'In my view this is the worst thing you can suggest to someone with cancer.' However, women are traditional targets for blame. How sad to add to women's guilt by making them feel they became sick because they weren't strong enough or wise enough to resist cancer.

Despite the lack of consensus about breast cancer, there do seem to be a number of 'risk factors'. Most of these influence the hormonal environment of a woman's body. Many are linked with the female hormone, oestrogen.

Risk factors

Diet seems to be a key cause of breast cancer. There is mounting evidence that the foods we eat – or don't eat – are linked to the development of cancer.

In evolutionary terms, the 'natural' state for human beings is 'to be hungry', says Julian Peto, Professor of Epidemiology at the Institute of Cancer Research. Our ancestors, he argues, spent their time running around, being hungry – especially during winter. They also breastfed their babies.

Various studies show that the more animal fat we eat, the higher the risk of breast cancer. Being overweight is also linked with breast cancer in post-menopausal women. This could be because fat cells release oestrogen, which has a role in breast cancer.

A study from the European Institute of Oncology in Milan (*Independent*, autumn 1992) showed that girls who eat a low-calorie diet during puberty may be at a lower risk of developing breast cancer in later life.

However, other studies contradict these findings. 'We've found no association between a high fat intake and the risk of breast cancer,' says Professor Walter Willett of the Harvard School of Public Health (*Observer*, 19.7.92). The same study found that women who actively reduce their intake of fat might also be increasing their risk of breast cancer.

As with other breast disorders, it seems that our Western **pattern of childbearing** and **breastfeeding** may be implicated in breast cancer. In short, the more periods you have in your life, the higher your risk of breast cancer. Women who start their periods early, have few babies comparatively late in life – or none at all – and who have a late menopause are more likely to develop breast cancer. Having children early – in your teens or early twenties – seems to have a protective effect.

According to an American researcher Dr Paul Mills (*Observer*, 19.7.92):

> A typical Eastern female doesn't start menstruating until 16 or 17. She'll marry and have her first pregnancy in her late teens, breast-feed for a long time (to prevent conception as well as ensuring the baby's health), then go on to have several more pregnancies. She's also lean, working hard on a low-calorie, low-fat diet. By contrast, the average age of menarche in the US is 12.8 and getting younger. A typical female will delay having her two children until she's 25 to 30, breastfeeding is less common, and she may be overweight.

Over the years there have also been many studies on the effect of **the Pill** on breast cancer. It is now widely accepted that the Pill does have a small effect on the breast cancer risks of young women. For women under thirty-five, the risk goes up from one in 500 to one in 300.

It could be that the Pill may speed up a cancer which is already there. Doctors will point out that these slight risks have to be weighed against the risk of an unwanted pregnancy.

There does seem to be a link between **HRT** (artificial hormones given to lessen unpleasant symptoms of the menopause) and breast cancer. 'The risk of breast cancer is increased by 30 per cent in women who have taken it for eight years or more,' says Judy Deacon. We don't know yet what the long-term effects are if women go on taking HRT, however the risks diminish when women stop taking it.

HRT and breast cancer are both common in the same sort of age-group, and they may often coincide without a link between them. Women who want to start on HRT would be wise to have a breast examination first, and to discuss the pros and cons of HRT with their GP, especially if they have a family history of the disease. As with the Pill, it makes sense to balance any possible risks of HRT against the risks of the conditions it prevents – like osteoporosis and heart disease. As Julian Peto put it, in general terms, HRT 'can cause breast cancer but protects against everything else'.

The question of whether **alcohol** can cause breast cancer is as yet unresolved. Some scientists believe that even three drinks a day (three half-pints of beer, glasses of wine, measures of spirits) may have an effect. And the younger you are when you drink, the greater the risk seems to be.

But stress is a factor in health, and if a glass of wine helps you to relax from time to time, so much the better. Penny Brohn, one of the founders of the Bristol Cancer Help Centre, was determined to beat her own breast cancer through alternative therapies, but still allowed herself a glass or two of wine a day for its 'stress-reducing, pleasure element'.

Large doses of high-energy, ionizing **radiation** – of the type produced by medical X-rays and by nuclear bombs – are known to increase the risk of breast cancer. For instance, the survivors of Hiroshima and Nagasaki experienced higher rates of cancer, including breast cancer.

Radiotherapy – part of the conventional treatment of cancer – uses controlled doses of ionizing radiation to kill cancer cells. Some researchers have argued that there may be a very small risk of developing cancer as a result of the treatment itself, but doctors believe that the benefits of the treatment are greater than the risks.

More controversial are the risks of low-energy radiation of the type which emanates from computer and TV screens. This is far less likely to damage cell structures, but there are unresolved questions about whether long-term exposure to low energy radiation may be dangerous, too.

Age is also an important factor in breast cancer. Old age is not a cause of the disease – women tend to get the disease after their thirties – but breast cancer risk does increase with age. Most cancers do develop slowly, and it could be that the 'cause' happens earlier in life, to be triggered into action as we get older.

Youth is a factor in breast cancer, too, because the developing breasts of young women seem to be especially sensitive to cancer-causing agents, like radiation.

There is an important family element in breast cancer. If your mother, aunt or sister has had breast cancer, then you too have an increased risk of the disease. Of the 25,000 cases of breast cancer in this country every year, about 1,250 (i.e. 5 per cent) are due to **genetic inheritance**.

Women with breast cancer in their families tend to suffer from anxiety about their own health, but it should be emphasized that only those women with at least two affected relatives under fifty years of age, are at much increased risk. Even then, the chances of not getting the disease are still good.

Can breast cancer be prevented?

What then can we do to protect ourselves against breast cancer? As you can see from the risk factors above, there is no single answer and no simple solution. But, says Judy Deacon, the best advice is 'to lead a healthy lifestyle and avoid getting fat'.

Current thinking is that a low-fat diet will cut down your risks, as will reducing obesity. A healthy diet may not be the answer to how to avoid breast cancer, but at least it can't do any harm and should improve your well-being.

What of our childbearing patterns? It's hardly likely that Western women are going to start giving birth in their teens in order to ward off breast cancer. On the other hand, there is one simple and natural way for women who do have children to give their bodies a rest from the many hundreds of periods we normally have across our lifetimes. Take the opportunity of motherhood to breastfeed fully and for as long as possible. It will not only benefit your baby, it may benefit you in more ways than you realize. A study in the *British Medical Journal* (July 1993) has indicated that breastfeeding for three months or longer can protect a woman against breast cancer. It also suggests that the more babies a woman breastfeeds the less likely she is to develop the disease.

A crucial tactic in combating cancer is to go to your doctor as soon as you notice any signs of a suspicious change in your breasts. The earlier you discover breast cancer, the better your chances of recovery.

Yet still we avoid examining ourselves and still we delay taking breast symptoms to our GPs. Eight thousand British women a year don't get medical treatment until their breast cancers are already advanced. A survey by the Cardiff Breast Clinic showed that 70 per cent of women with lumps in their breasts had delayed taking their symptoms to a family doctor. The delays varied from a few months to several years. The Cardiff survey found that most women who delayed going to a doctor feared hearing the cancer diagnosis.

We also learn from childhood that we are not supposed to expose our breasts except for sex. That makes it difficult for women to take their tops off in front of GPs and to submit to being looked at and touched.

Cancer experts talk in exasperated tones of British women's 'modesty' when it comes to breast symptoms. The word 'irrational' comes up a lot in the literature. Yet many of us know – from our own experiences and from friends – that GPs can be very dismissive of breast symptoms. Callers to the Breast Care Campaign's helpline frequently said their doctors were unsympathetic and that they were made to feel that they were wasting the doctor's time.

America is a country which has more breast cancer cases than we do – and yet fewer deaths. Barry Gusterson, Professor of Histopathology at the Institute of Cancer Research, thinks this is because the US is a 'screening-type society'.

How could we improve our survival rates from breast cancer? Apart from maintaining a good diet, Gusterson believes that 'changing cultural attitudes' could make a bigger difference than doctors. A change in cultural attitudes could encourage women to come forward earlier for treatment, so saving many lives.

There is also a possibility that the drug tamoxifen may one day be used to prevent breast cancer by blocking the hormone stimulation which breast cancers need to develop in the first place. (For more on tamoxifen, see Chapter Eleven.)

Screening for breast cancer

By the mid-1980s, the government was under pressure to do something about the mounting epidemic of breast cancer in this country. Other countries had already proved that a screening programme could protect lives. Professor Sir Patrick Forrest was appointed to head a working party to investigate the issue.

As a result of his report, the government announced in 1987 that it would set up a national network of breast screening centres to screen women aged fifty to sixty-five. The official prediction was that 1,250 women a year would be successfully treated for breast cancer as a result of the programme.

But why not younger women? (Women under fifty can be screened, but they must either get a referral from their GP, or they must go privately.) The reasons are mostly technical. Younger women have more glandular breast tissue than older women. This tissue is denser and shows up as white on a mammogram. Breast cancers also show up as white blobs, making them harder to spot in younger women.

There have been dissenting voices. Some women have argued that screening can falsely raise a woman's hope of a cure, when in reality all that is achieved is to tell her the bad news sooner rather than later. (However, there is no doubt that screening the over-fifties saves the lives of 20 per cent of women with breast cancer in this age group.)

There is also an argument that screening detects 'pre-cancers' or tiny tumours which might in due course have disappeared (dealt with by the immune system), so avoiding unnecessary stress and treatment. Microscopic tumours probably come and go anyway for much of our lives. The only advantage of spotting these would be to warn us to change our lifestyle to avoid any further damage to health.

Some women have also asked whether breast screening is worth it, given the inconvenience, anxiety and discomfort that the process can inflict. There are also questions about the safety of mammography, which repeatedly exposes the breast to radiation, a known cause of breast cancer.

Those who defend it say that screening definitely saves women's lives. They argue that doses of radiation are so low that they cannot cause harm. And it has been shown that mammography can pick up very small tumours. If these are treated quickly – before there is evidence of lymph node involvement – a woman's chances are much improved. At least 80 per cent of women in this category survive for at least ten years after treatment.

A further area of debate over screening concerns its timing. Currently, women eligible for screening are checked once every three years. But some specialists are concerned that this is too long a gap. Dr Ruth Warren, a radiologist in charge of screening at St Margaret's Hospital in Epping (*Horizon*, 6.1.92) believes:

> This is actually a financial issue. If you reduce the screening interval it will cost the government more . . . I think many people who work with breast cancer might prefer the interval to be a little shorter than two years, in that we would then see more of the aggressive tumours at small size.

Meanwhile at least a third of the women who are invited to attend screening refuse the invitation.

What we can prevent . . .

It is hard to face the fear of breast cancer. We don't yet know what causes it, we can't prevent it and we can't 'cure' it.

But there are things we can prevent. We can prevent our own ignorance by finding out all we can about this disease. We can try to prevent the distress that follows unsympathetic treatment by asking questions and making choices. And we can improve our chances of survival by acting quickly if we suspect a breast problem.

11
Breast cancer:
dealing with the reality

Time to act

You may have noticed it yourself. It may have first shown up on
a mammogram. But the shadow of breast cancer is now in your
life. What do you do?

Go to your doctor straight away. Don't wait until the children
go back to school/the job you are working on is over/you have
more time (reasons women often give for delaying).

Acting quickly could save your life – and could save you from
extra surgery, too. Doctors claim that breast cancer can be
stopped in its tracks, if it is caught in its earliest stages. Two-
thirds of women whose breast cancers are detected by screening
can be successfully treated, as can a quarter of women who go
to a doctor with a lump.

According to Ian Fentiman of the Imperial Cancer Research
Fund:

> Women with breast cancers up to one centimetre in diameter, with
> no spread to the lymph glands under the arm, live as long as
> women who don't have breast cancer. (*Guardian*, 20.10.92)

Finding out

There are two main routes to a breast cancer diagnosis. One is through the National Breast Screening Programme, and the other is through your local health service in the form of your GP (or Well Woman Clinic or Family Planning Clinic).

Whatever route you follow, do try to take your partner or a friend or relative along with you to your medical appointments. These can be very stressful, especially if you are waiting to hear a diagnosis. Emotional and moral support in these circumstances can make a lot of difference, and you may want your companion to act as your 'advocate' – asking questions or speaking for you – as your treatment gets under way.

It may be a good idea to take a tape recorder to medical appointments, too (or ask your companion to do this). A recording can help a woman to recall the details of what the doctor has said, so often forgotten in the stress of the moment. It can also help her to break the news to her family, who will want to know what is likely to happen. These days some hospitals have begun to provide such tape recordings for women patients. Increasingly they also have a specialist breast nurse present, ready to give emotional and practical support to newly diagnosed women.

Finding out through screening

Many women (aged fifty plus) have their first encounter with the prospect of cancer when they get a letter from the National Breast Screening Programme inviting them to attend a clinic.

This may be in a mobile unit – often more convenient for women in rural areas – or it may be in a static unit which is part of a hospital.

Wherever it may be, the national programme claims to have the best service of its kind in the world, and women can be sure of meeting with specialist staff with first-rate equipment at their disposal. Every screening centre must have a specialist surgeon attached, and according to Julietta Patnick, who heads the programme:

> We try to make the clinics as attractive as possible; we try to cut down on waiting; and we remember at all times that we are dealing with healthy women.

Unjustly, women who are not invited for screening (i.e. women under fifty and women who find their own breast lumps) cannot use these facilities, a situation that calls for change.

At the screening appointment, a woman is given a mammogram, in which the breasts are compressed between metal plates and X-ray photographs taken of them. The appointment should take no more than half an hour. Most women will get a letter within a few weeks saying that all is well and their next visit will be in three years' time.

However, around 7 per cent of women are asked to go back for another mammogram. They may also have a physical examination of the breasts. They may have an ultrasound scan which can show whether a suspicious lump is fluid-filled – in which case it is likely to be a cyst – or if the lump is solid, which means it could be cancer or some other form of breast disorder. They may have fine needle aspiration cytology, a kind of biopsy in which a small sample of a lump can be taken through a needle (usually without anaesthetic) and then examined for signs of cancer.

Most of this group of recalled women will also discover that their breast lump is harmless. One woman in every hundred who goes for screening, however, will find that their doctor is not happy with their screening results. The next step is an open biopsy, an operation to take a sample of breast tissue which is done under a general anaesthetic. This is not a major operation; it may involve an overnight stay in hospital, it may be done on a day basis. At this stage a woman has a fifty/fifty chance of being told that she has cancer.

If she is diagnosed as having cancer, she can then choose where she wants to be treated. Often women choose to stay with the surgeon who did their original biopsy, as they have an established contact.

Finding out by the local route

Women who find a breast lump or other symptom themselves will usually make an appointment with their GP (or Family Planning or Well Woman Clinic). Usually, a GP will refer women on to the breast clinic of a hospital, which may or may not have a specialist surgeon, depending on where she lives. There could be a two-week gap before the next appointment, when women are examined by a surgeon (or one of his or her team) and questioned about their medical history, including any family history of breast disease.

Usually, the next step is a mammogram – which means another appointment and more waiting – followed by waiting for another appointment in order to get the results. (All this waiting can be extremely stressful, not to say galling, in the light of medical advice that women should have symptoms seen to without delay.)

If a lump is found or confirmed, the surgeon will want to do a biopsy before recommending treatment. Again, do try to have someone with you on these occasions to give you emotional support and practical help.

Asking for the best

For any woman newly diagnosed with breast cancer, a vitally important question to ask is, 'Will I be cared for by specialists?' But many of us never ask this question, because we are too upset or too intimidated or too polite – and because we are not expected to ask for the best for ourselves. As Andrea Whalley, former director of Breast Cancer Care puts it;

> This is one of the most important questions a woman can ask. But it's rather like asking, 'Will you use a condom?' It takes tremendous confidence to ask on your own behalf.

This is a time when a sister or a partner or supportive friend can usefully step in as an advocate to ask the questions we find hard to ask for ourselves.

Ideally every woman with breast cancer should have specialist care. Andrea Whalley argues:

> Increasingly it is recognized that women should have access to team care, including breast care nurses, oncologists, surgeons and radiologists, all of whom are specialists in breast cancer. Such a team can diagnose and manage the disease, taking you every step

of the way and discussing every step with each other – and with their patients. In this approach you have a number of brains all coming from different specialisms, all working on what is best for you, rather than one general surgeon who may have a single and unbending idea of how to treat the disease.

If you (or your advocate) want to make sure you are getting first-rate treatment, the answer should be 'yes' to most of the following questions:

- Has your surgeon performed regular breast operations in the past year and taken a special interest in breast cancer? (This makes sure you have an expert operating on your breasts.)
- Is your hospital involved in clinical trials? (If it is, you may have an opportunity to try new drugs or treatments not otherwise available.)
- Do those treating you have access to the latest equipment, such as ultrasound scanning machines and fine needle aspiration cytology?
- Is there a breast care nurse available as a part of your health care? (Breast care nurses are crucial to recovery, in providing information and support.)

If you have any doubts about your diagnosis or about your proposed treatments, ask for a second opinion (or your advocate could ask). It is well known that in this country treatment is mostly a matter of pot luck and where you live. Women who are fortunate enough to live near a hospital with specialist staff may get the best and the latest treatments, while those who don't may be treated by general surgeons with little expertise who perform mastectomies as a matter of course.

To add to the confusion there is no consensus about treatments, even amongst the experts. Under the circumstances, asking for a second opinion is a very reasonable request. (You have no legal right to a second opinion, but in practice, very few doctors refuse.)

Who is 'the best'?

The next obvious question is, 'Where (and who) are the best doctors?' It is not a question that anyone working in the breast cancer field wants to answer for fear of alienating the medical establishment. This is widely regarded as a 'political' question much to be avoided – although many in the field are keen for someone else to come up with the answers! There is also an understandable fear that anyone identified as being 'the best' would be swamped with patients.

Nor is it a question that can be accurately answered: in the absence of a consensus about breast cancer, 'best' care is still a matter of opinion. Nor is it possible, without any national database of information about treatments, to come up with a definitive list of 'best' doctors or 'best' treatments.

However, it is valid to ask whether your hospital is one of the acknowledged centres of excellence in breast cancer. While stressing again that no list is comprehensive, the hospitals that are thought to be amongst the best by Professor Robert Mansel (Senior Lecturer and Consultant Surgeon at the University of Wales College of Medicine, member of the London Cancer Review Group and secretary of the Surgical Research Society) include:

• Christie Hospital, Manchester
• City Hospital, Nottingham

- Glasgow Western Infirmary
- Guy's Hospital, London
- Leeds General Infirmary
- Newcastle General Hospital
- Ninewells Hospital, Dundee
- Royal County Hospital, Guildford
- Royal Infirmary, Huddersfield
- Royal Liverpool Hospital
- Royal Marsden Hospital, London and Sutton
- Selly Oak Hospital, Birmingham
- University Hospital of Wales, Cardiff
- Western Infirmary, Edinburgh

There are other ways of checking whether your hospital or surgeon ranks highly in terms of expertise. One way, suggests Julietta Patnick, is to ask to be treated by a surgeon who is linked to the national screening programme and who is therefore likely to be an experienced specialist.

If you are diagnosed through the screening programme you will have access to such a specialist. If you are diagnosed through the local GP route, you can ask your GP to refer you to a surgeon associated with the screening programme. Julietta Patnick does stress, however, that the programme does not have a monopoly on good doctors.

What happens if you don't live near any of these centres of excellence or near a specialist surgeon, but want to be treated by one? Much depends on whether your health authority will pay for you to go to a different area for treatment. It can take a great deal of confidence, not to mention string-pulling, to get treatment anywhere else.

In practice, most women are treated at their nearest hospital, sometimes for reasons of convenience, sometimes because they are not aware of the alternatives. And since the restructuring of the NHS women are finding they have less choice in places of treatment because of financial constraints.

Questions of care

There is no single treatment for breast cancer. This is a capricious disease which has more than twenty forms, and every woman's treatment will depend on many factors, such as the size, spread and type of cancer, and the age, general health and wishes of the woman.

None the less, once the cancer diagnosis has been confirmed, you are likely to have questions for your surgeon. (Some women prefer to leave everything in the hands of their doctors without asking any questions, and this is equally their right.)

But the chances are that, having just been knocked flat by the news, you don't feel strong enough to ask questions. Again, this is a time that your 'advocate' can step in to do the asking for you.

For instance, you may want to know:

- How large is the cancer?
- How far has it spread?
- Where exactly is the cancer?
- What type of cancer is it?
- Will a mastectomy be necessary? If so, why? (Having a mastectomy doesn't necessarily mean the cancer is 'worse'.)
- Are more conservative treatments – like lumpectomy – available?
- Is breast reconstruction available after an operation? (Ask

about this before a mastectomy or lumpectomy: it could make a difference to your surgery.)

• Will I need any other follow-up treatments, such as radiotherapy, chemotherapy or hormone therapy?

Some women will want to know, 'How long will I live?' This is not a question that doctors will want to answer because they cannot give an accurate prediction. But Frank Arnold, a surgeon in Manchester, puts it like this:

> The disease can be slow-growing in the old, who often die of unrelated 'natural' causes first. In younger women, 35 to 50 per cent will die within 10 years. Many of the rest will have a normal life expectancy. Identifying those women who would do badly, in order to offer them a choice of aggressive treatments, is something we are not very good at. (*Independent*, 4.12.90)

You may also want to know if your treatment is part of a trial. Because doctors are undecided about the most effective treatments, trials are being conducted to compare the different options in different areas. Five per cent of cancer patients in this country are being given the option of taking part in trials. You do not have to take part, but if you choose to, you should be fully informed of all its aspects.

A useful leaflet on your rights, and questions you should ask (such as 'What is the reason for the trial?' and 'What will happen if I say no?'), is available from Consumers for Ethics in Research, P O Box 1365, London N16 OBW.

You also have the right to ask for time to think before agreeing on treatments with your surgeon. A few days or even weeks will make little difference to the disease, but they could make a lot of difference to your future health and emotional state.

The medical profession in this country is extremely secretive with the information it holds about patients. From the time your

GP gives you your first sealed letter of referral to take to the hospital (many a woman has rushed home to steam it open), your doctor's written opinions about your illness are likely to be kept from you.

For instance, all the information about what kind of cancer you have will be in your biopsy report, which is not shown to you. In their book *Disorderly Breasts*, Sarah Boston and Jill Louw suggest that you ask to see your report:

> if only to see and check the evidence for yourself. One woman, years after a mastectomy, still harboured a lingering doubt expressed in the words, 'I never saw the biopsy report. Perhaps . . .' If reading the biopsy report dispels doubts, ask to see it and, if you don't understand the language, ask to have it explained.

It is high time the medical profession were more open with us. The Europa Donna campaign, launched in 1992 by the European School of Oncology in Milan to improve breast care in Europe, calls on all specialists to:

- Explain with professional care each patient's case, ensuring that she has thoroughly understood.
- Allow the patient to see her case history whenever possible and consult with other specialists involved.

Choices in treatment

Conventional medicine has three basic strategies in treating breast cancer, which can be used alone or in combination with each other. These are surgery, radiotherapy and drugs (chemotherapy and hormone therapy). The kind of treatment a doctor will suggest depends on a range of factors, including the tumour (its type, size and whether it has spread), a woman's age and health, and the doctor's attitude to treatments.

Most women with breast cancer (80 per cent) have some form of surgery, either to remove the breast or the lump in the breast. The other therapies are often used after an operation for breast cancer, or they can be offered instead of surgery. Increasingly, women are drawing on complementary therapies in addition to conventional methods, and many hospitals now encourage this approach. Only a tiny minority opt out of conventional care altogether.

Remember that while your doctor can recommend treatments, and should discuss the options thoroughly with you, the choice remains yours. Doctors cannot predict with certainty what will happen as a result of treatment, and different doctors have different views on treatments. Nor can a doctor operate without your written consent. If you have unresolved doubts, ask for a second opinion (it may not be a different opinion), or contact one of the helping organizations listed at the back of this book.

Surgery

Breast cancer operations involve either the removal of the breast (**mastectomy**), or of the lump and some surrounding tissue from the breast (**lumpectomy**).

Mastectomy generally leaves women with a flat area where the breast used to be and a scar across its centre. Lumpectomy generally leaves a dent in the breast plus a scar. A lumpectomy that takes away a larger section of breast tissue is called **segmentectomy**, and this leaves a larger dent.

In the past women commonly had **radical mastectomies** for breast cancer, in which muscles from the chest wall would be removed as well as the breast. But the more radical the surgery, the more a woman is likely to suffer after the operation – emotionally as well as physically – and radical mastectomies are now rare. However, some women are still advised to have a **modified radical mastectomy** which takes away the breast together with a small chest muscle and the lymph nodes. (In most breast cancer operations the surgeon will either remove the lymph glands from under the arm or take a few glands out to assess whether the cancer has spread.)

These days, smaller and more 'conservative' (in the sense of conserving the breast) operations are more common. Several studies have shown that women recover from breast cancer just as well after conservative treatments as they do after mastectomy. According to the 1986 King's Fund Forum on breast cancer:

> There is no evidence that mastectomy or more extensive surgery, as opposed to local removal of the tumour, leads to longer survival. The risk of local recurrence is greater with breast conservation. However, this risk can be reduced substantially by radiotherapy.

Sometimes however, doctors do advise that mastectomy is the best option. This could be because the breast is small, or the lump is directly behind the nipple, or the cancer is an 'aggressive' type. And sometimes women choose mastectomy because they don't want to live with the fear that the cancer might recur in that breast.

Premenopausal women may benefit from controversial new research at Guy's Hospital in London which found that women who had operations in the second half of their menstrual cycle

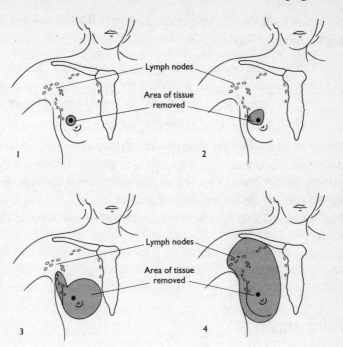

Figure 11: **1 Lumpectomy**. Only the lump is removed, together with some normal surrounding tissue.

2 Segmentectomy. A larger section of breast tissue is removed with the lump.

3 Simple mastectomy. All the breast tissue is removed, but the muscles of the breast are left intact.

4 Modified radical mastectomy. All the breast tissue, the under-arm lymph nodes and the lining over the chest muscles are removed.

Lymph nodes: These are likely to be removed completely or for sampling. The condition of the lymph nodes is an important indicator of how far the disease has spread and whether further treatment is necessary.

Reproduced by kind permission of the Royal Marsden Hospital: copyright 1991. Taken from 'Cancer of the Breast', Patient Information Series.

did better than those operated on in the first half. According to Ian Fentiman of Guy's:

> Of those we operated on at the 'safe' time, in the second half of the cycle, something like 80 per cent were alive and well ten years later – as against something like 50 per cent of those we operated on at the 'unsafe' time. (*Horizon*, 6.1.92)

Fentiman estimates that changing the timing of women's operations could save some 600 lives a year in Britain. Unfortunately, other hospitals haven't been able to confirm these findings, but there is no reason why women shouldn't ask to be operated on later in their cycle – until we know for sure one way or the other.

After surgery

After surgery women are likely to have some pain or discomfort, as well as a drainage tube in the wound for a few days. Stitches are usually removed about ten days after the operation.

The length of the stay in hospital will depend on the kind of operation. Women who have had mastectomies don't usually go home for about eight or ten days, whereas women who have had lumpectomies or segmentectomies may go home after only a few days. If you are in pain, do let the nurse looking after you know, and ask for effective painkillers.

After a mastectomy women are usually given an artificial breast or prosthesis to wear inside a bra. This is made of lightweight, foam material and can protect the tender area after the operation. There are various types of prosthesis supplied without charge by the NHS. For more information contact Breast Cancer Care, which has its own prosthesis fitting service.

It may be possible to have a breast reconstruction at the same time as a mastectomy, or some months – even years – afterwards. If possible, discuss the option of breast reconstruction with the surgeon at the beginning of treatment. Other women prefer not to wear a prosthesis and not to have reconstruction (see page 236).

When women have had lymph nodes removed from the armpit, or have had radiotherapy to the armpit, there can be a risk of lymphoedema. This happens when lymphatic fluid flows to the hand or arm in response to any sort of injury, and then fails to drain away. The swelling that results can be very sore. BACUP has a useful leaflet on lymphoedema.

How will I look? How will I feel?

The experience of breast cancer can be extremely traumatic for women, and one of the greatest worries is that of being disfigured by surgery. Our breasts are deeply important to our sense of being a woman, to our self-image, sexuality and self-confidence. The loss of a breast or part of a breast is often felt as a bereavement – and it can take a long time for a woman to come to terms with her loss.

How then does a woman approach the moment of looking at her scar after surgery? Alone? With her partner? In the company of a nurse?

Every woman needs to make that decision for herself, but the organization Breast Cancer Care does recommend that women take a look at their scars before leaving hospital, giving themselves time to come to terms with their changed appearance. Whichever strategy women choose to help them cope, the months after breast surgery are often a time of devastating and conflicting emotions, ranging from grief and anger to relief that the cancer has been treated.

In the past, women often went through these traumas alone, but today, changing attitudes and a network of organizations concerned with breast cancer have made support available to those who look for it. BACUP has a face-to-face cancer counselling service in London and can put women in touch with trained counsellors in their local area who will offer support at any time during or after treatment. Breast Cancer Care also has a nationwide volunteer support programme and it puts women in touch with others who have had cancer so that they can share experiences and offer mutual support.

And of course, a loving partner or friend, together with a specially trained breast nurse or sympathetic doctor, can make an enormous difference to how a woman gets through the experience of breast cancer.

Radiotherapy

Radiotherapy is a form of treatment which uses radiation to 'burn out' any cancer cells which may have been left behind after a mastectomy, lumpectomy or segmentectomy. Sometimes radiotherapy is the sole form of treatment used for breast cancer; sometimes it is a treatment for a cancer which has reappeared in the breast.

After a few visits to the radiotherapy department of the hospital to plan your treatment, doctors will draw marks on your skin to show which area of your body is to be treated. Treatment normally takes place for five days a week over about a four week period and is quite painless.

Each treatment lasts only a few minutes, during which you lie still, as if you were having an X-ray. You will be alone in the treatment room, but you will be able to talk to your radiographer who will be watching from the next room.

This kind of radiotherapy is called 'external radiotherapy' and it does not make you radioactive. However women who have had lumpectomies or segmentectomies are sometimes given 'internal radiotherapy', a kind of treatment in which radioactive wires are implanted into the breast under anaesthetic. As soon as the wires are removed, all radioactivity is removed too – but until then there are restrictions on the amount of time you can spend with other people.

Both kinds of radiotherapy can have upsetting side-effects. Sometimes the skin becomes red and 'weepy', and some women suffer nausea and tiredness.

As with so many other aspects of breast cancer, debate still rages on the effectiveness and safety of radiotherapy. Doubts centre on the wisdom of using an agent which can in itself cause cancer to 'cure' cancer, and this treatment can have long-term effects on other tissues in the target area.

However, most doctors argue that the risks are very minor compared to the benefits. Radiation can be very effective in treating breast cancer, and it can also shrink secondary tumours and alleviate pain.

Chemotherapy

Chemotherapy is the use of anti-cancer (cytotoxic) drugs to destroy cancer cells which may be left in your body after surgery or radiotherapy. It treats the whole body by attacking cancer cells wherever they have travelled to from the breast, but unfortunately, healthy cells also get damaged in the process.

The drugs are usually injected into a vein, but they may be given by mouth. The course of treatment usually lasts a few days, but because they make you more vulnerable to infection, your body will take a few weeks to recover from any side-effects. You may have chemotherapy as an out-patient, but sometimes chemotherapy requires a few days in hospital.

Like radiotherapy, chemotherapy is used as a precautionary measure against stray cancer cells. It is also used to treat any recurrence of cancer. And like radiotherapy it has its opponents and its defenders. The arguments go on: when should it be used? At what stage? How effective is it?

According to Richard Peto of the Imperial Cancer Research Fund (*Horizon* 6.1.92):

> Doctors really are reluctant to accept widespread use of chemotherapy and there will always be a balance between whether the difference in survival is actually worth the side-effects.

But a ten-year study of 75,000 women by Peto, published in *Lancet* (December, 1991), showed that chemotherapy together with hormonal treatments of breast cancer could save 10,000 lives a year worldwide. For every thousand women treated this way, up to 120 will be alive ten years later who would otherwise have died. The best results came from using a combination of chemotherapy and tamoxifen.

Another kind of chemotherapy, 'neo-adjuvant' therapy, takes place before surgery. Doctors claim that this can shrink tumours, minimizing surgery, and may also 'sterilize' the tumour, so preventing its spread during surgery.

Chemotherapy often gets bad press because it can have some very nasty side-effects including loss of hair, vomiting and diarrhoea, mouth ulcers and general debilitation. These days however, anti-sickness drugs are available to counteract any nausea. Some fortunate people have no side-effects at all, and all side-effects do cease as treatment ends. (BACUP has free booklets on chemotherapy and on coping with hair loss.)

Hormone therapy

Like radiotherapy and chemotherapy, hormone therapy can be recommended to those (usually post-menopausal women) being treated for breast cancer.

The female hormones oestrogen and progesterone (which occur naturally in our bodies) can influence the growth of breast cancer cells. Hormone therapy, which is in fact anti-hormone treatment, stops the natural female hormones from encouraging breast cancers to grow.

Tamoxifen is the commonest form of hormone treatment (taken by mouth in tablet form) and a course can last from several months to several years. Its side-effects are few, although it can stop periods and cause early menopause in younger women.

Tamoxifen, originally designed as a contraceptive, is now thought to be the best treatment to improve the survival chances

of post-menopausal women. In women whose tumours are sensitive to hormones, tamoxifen blocks the oestrogen receptors
on the breast cancer cell, with the effect of stopping the growth
of malignant cells which are dependent on oestrogen for
growth.

Tamoxifen is not a new discovery. Doctors have been using it
since 1971. But only recently have they realized its potential. In
a Cancer Research Campaign study, tamoxifen reduced the risk
of further tumours in women with breast cancer by 40 per cent.
It also reduced the risk of a cancer recurring in the same place
by 20 per cent.

To test this finding in healthy women at increased risk of
developing a breast cancer because of their family history, a
double-blind trial was set up. Women were told they would
either get tamoxifen or a placebo (a blank sample used in
medical testing which has no physical effect. No one but the
computer would know who was on tamoxifen and who was on
the placebo. Scientists hoped that after eight years, the women
taking tamoxifen would have fewer breast cancers, showing that
the drug can prevent the disease.

However, the trial has raised difficult ethical questions. Is it
right to give thousands of healthy women a powerful and
potentially toxic drug?

Despite evidence that tamoxifen has some beneficial side-effects
(it reduces the risk of heart disease by lowering cholesterol), the
trial has been delayed while the Medical Research Council looked
more closely into its ethics. The slight possibility that tamoxifen
could increase other tumours (like cancer of the uterus) also has
to be resolved.

To date, there is no tamoxifen trial in the UK, but the FDA in
America has approved a big tamoxifen study and there is also a
study going on in Italy. In the US, any woman over sixty can

join the trial, as can any woman from a 'high risk' family (women with at least two close relatives under fifty who have had the disease).

As for the future, Professor Barry Gusterson believes the way forward in breast cancer research could be to produce a contraceptive pill which also prevents the disease. 'Drug companies', he says, 'are working on this idea at the moment. But it remains a distant hope.'

The role of the breast care nurse

As women have testified many times in this book, having access to a breast care nurse can be very important in a woman's recovery from cancer.

A breast care nurse is a nurse who, on top of her general training, has taken an advanced course in the care of women with breast cancer. She may also have had extra training in counselling.

Her work involves caring for and supporting women with breast cancer from the time of diagnosis, throughout their treatment and during the time that they are recovering. A breast care nurse can answer questions about breast cancer, as well as acting as a source of information and – where needed – as a 'patient advocate'. She also teaches nurses and doctors about breast cancer, and keeps up with the latest in breast cancer research.

A breast care nurse can also fit prostheses and advise about breast reconstruction. She may run a clinic and/or support group for women with lymphoedema (swelling of the arm caused by removal of the lymph glands), and is well placed to put women with breast cancer in touch with the network of volunteers who have been through the same experience.

Breast care nurses are attached to hospital-based breast care teams, which means that they are available to women who have been referred to a hospital by their GP. There are now some 170 breast care nurses in the UK (in 1980 there were only three), and – fortunately for women – their numbers are still increasing.

Having your say

Sadly, the reality of breast cancer for most women is still a frightening and life-threatening ordeal. We are still far from understanding this disease and far from tackling it with the urgency that women deserve.

But there have been some improvements in treatments in recent years. A breast cancer diagnosis no longer means automatic disfigurement through radical mastectomy. Increasingly, surgeons are recognizing that women feel strongly about their breasts, and that the more conservative options such as lumpectomy can be just as effective.

The advent of tamoxifen has halved the recurrence of breast cancer in older women. The more recent chemotherapy cocktails have fewer nasty side-effects and have also improved survival rates. Radiotherapy techniques are improving too. We also have a national screening programme in place.

We still can't tell what causes this disease. We still can't prevent it. We still can't bring the death rate down. But we can improve our chances by going to a doctor as soon as we notice symptoms, and we can take up invitations to screenings.

We can also do something about the emotional devastation of a breast cancer diagnosis. Research shows that women with this disease suffer less from anxiety and depression when they have a say in the decisions about their treatments. And increasingly when it comes to breast cancer, women are making themselves heard.

12
Choosing complementary care: alternatives in treatment

Millions of women the world over have now been helped by conventional medical treatments. Most of us would not be without them: the appalling agonies women went through before modern treatments and anaesthesia hardly bear thinking about. The very fact that so many women now question the role of conventional medicine and of doctors is a kind of testament to their achievements.

None the less, most women do question conventional medicine at some level. In earlier chapters this book examined how our breasts are seen in society. Women have described how their breasts are 'taken' from them by porn and pin-ups, treated as detached 'parts' by advertising and the media, fought over in the battle for breastfeeding. It is no coincidence that women talk about their medical experiences in the same terms: a common complaint is that we are expected to 'hand over' our breasts for treatment as if they don't belong to us.

This issue of 'whose breasts are they?' crops up in relation to conventional medicine just as it crops up in relation to fashion, to breastfeeding, to men. Are we to have responsibility for and control over our own bodies, or are we to give our breasts unquestioningly to doctors? Must we accept the hierarchies of the old-fashioned hospital, where doctors too often assume they know what is best for us, where women's views and feelings are often neglected and where the consultant is God? Or is there an alternative?

We have seen also that there is no consensus about the best medical treatments in breast cancer: it follows that some women feel the breast is a battleground for doctors, as they compete in an adversarial system for their own theories of best treatment.

Many women turn to complementary therapies (usually in addition to conventional medicine) as an option which treats them as a whole person, without separating breast from self. Many are looking, too, for a way of healing which involves them as people, requiring them to take some measure of responsibility and control – rather than behaving obediently and dependently.

Breast cancer rebels

The breast cancer literature features many rebellious women who braved the anger of the medical establishment when they rejected recommended treatments and took the 'alternative' path. Some of them are still alive; some of them are not. It is not possible to say whether complementary medicine helped them to live longer, but many say it has helped them to live better.

Penny Brohn, one of the founders of the Bristol Cancer Help Centre, is one long-surviving rebel. She believed her breast cancer was a disease of the whole person and she set out to find spiritual and emotional healing together with physical healing, rejecting conventional medicine until she had found her own way forward.

Much of her battle was to do with control over her own body. In her book *Gentle Giants*, she writes of how she watched women on her hospital ward being emotionally rewarded for being 'good' in accepting their doctors' verdicts:

> I saw them buying the comfort they needed with their compliance . . .
> (But) I had to operate on the darkness the experience exposed, not the experience itself.

When the photographer Jo Spence was diagnosed with breast cancer, she submitted herself – as she put it – to the 'medical machine' and had a lumpectomy operation (after refusing mastectomy). But before long, she was fighting to 'get off medical orthodoxy's production line'. As she wrote in her book, *Putting Myself in the Picture*:

> I was aware in my hospital bed, as I took the first steps towards defiance of the medical orthodoxy, that it would be a long and lonely confrontation. It took an immense amount of courage initially to say no, that I didn't want to be mutilated (beyond the three vivid slashes that now adorn my breast), or to be radiated or drugged.

Jo Spence began to eat healthily, following the eating guidelines of the Bristol Cancer Help Centre. She shed four stone of excess weight, sought out therapists, took up co-counselling and learned to be assertive. With a naturopath and psychiatric social worker she set out to work through her 'closed-off systems of logic [and] repressed desires'. Eventually, she opted for Traditional Chinese Medicine (TCM), in which the patient is encouraged to take some responsibility for getting and staying well:

> [TCM] means more work for the patient, and the necessity to make informed decisions; at its best, it means the shattering of lifelong habits in relation to food, drugs, exercise and breathing, and the awakening of the knowledge that the body cannot deal for

ever with a completely unharmonious relationship with the psychic, spiritual, social, economic, living and loving conditions. In plain English, I learned to love myself better and get more in touch with my actual needs and feelings so that I could start to try to change things wherever possible.

It sounds like a tall order, but Jo Spence (who died ten years after her cancer was diagnosed) clearly believed it was well worth while:

> It is my belief that TCM offers me the best chance of survival as a cancer patient, or at least a better quality of life. It does not pretend to offer me a 'cure', but is a way of managing the illness, putting it at bay and perhaps slowing it down.

Four years after starting TCM she wrote:

> Now I can begin to hear myself ticking over again. No miracles, no racing motor, no rejuvenated going off into the sunset . . . it's just that I can begin to hear my inner voices speaking to me in ways I didn't realize were possible.

Penny Brohn also found unexpected emotional and spiritual rewards in her personal battle with breast cancer. One night, early in her illness, she and her husband faced each other and communicated as they never had before:

> The indescribable sweetness and joy of that night and the peace that came from it was so beautiful a consequence of being hit by a virtually incurable disease that I can honestly say it was worth it.

Boosting immunity

Many people now believe that our immune systems can protect us against cancerous changes in our own cells throughout our lives. It could be that we all produce cancerous cells from time to time, and that our immune systems destroy these before they have the chance to take hold or spread – as long as we are in good health. But sometimes, when we are tired or low, our immune systems are weakened.

We all know that colds and flu can take hold at these times: it could be that cancer also takes hold when our resistance is low. Ageing weakens our immune systems, too, which could explain why cancer is so much a disease of old age. Conventional medical treatments – chiefly surgery, radiotherapy and drug therapies – also weaken our own healing processes at the same time as they weaken cancer.

Most alternative treatments are designed to strengthen our immune systems, helping our bodies to heal themselves. They are not 'miracle cures', but they can help us towards better health. Few of them can be scientifically 'proven', and scientists complain that the complementary practitioners won't submit their therapies to controlled trials.

Critics also point to the 'placebo effect', arguing that 30 per cent of people feel better for simply having been treated – even if they have only been given sugar pills. However, when it comes to breast cancer, it is clear that science doesn't have all the answers either.

Pioneering programme

One of the leading complementary health centres in Britain is the Bristol Cancer Help Centre, founded in 1980. Many leading NHS centres now incorporate aspects of the Bristol programme into their own treatments, most prominently the Hammersmith Hospital in London.

There was controversy over the Centre in recent years after a group of leading cancer specialists published the results of a study (September 1990) which suggested that women treated at the Centre were more likely to die of cancer – and to have their cancer recur – than women who had only conventional treatments.

In the furore and media attention that followed, the Centre faced accusations that their treatments were actually harming women with breast cancer.

Yet within months, this theory had been discredited and it was recognized that the report had not compared like with like: women going to the Bristol Centre tended to have more advanced breast cancer in the first place. It followed that women going to the Bristol Centre were closer to death anyway than women who were having only conventional treatments. Many leading doctors now believe that the Centre can help women with breast cancer to feel better – which can only be a good thing.

It was a serious setback for the Centre, but it has survived with its international reputation intact. In the 1990s it is continuing to improve its links with the NHS and also hoping for further, more accurate research into its achievements.

The Bristol Centre offers a wide range of therapies in its holistic treatment of cancer, including relaxation, meditation, visualization, dietary and art therapy, and counselling. The majority of people who draw on its services are women with breast cancer.

As a part of its therapeutic programme it aims to tackle the emotional, social and spiritual distress associated with the diagnosis of cancer. Much emphasis is placed on restoring peace of mind and a sense of control and purpose. In this way patients are helped to tap into their inner resources of self-healing and strength.

Treatment is not free of charge. A five-day residential course typically costs £495. But no one is refused a place because they can't pay; there is a bursary fund to help with fees, and the Department of Social Security may also help people who are receiving benefit. The one-day introductory course costs £50 and there are also one-day follow-up courses.

The Bristol Centre does not claim to be an alternative to medical treatment – few practitioners of complementary medicine do – and it is rare for women to take the road of rejecting medical treatments altogether.

Eating for health

A keystone of many complementary therapies – from homeopathy to herbalism – is diet. But many so-called 'cancer diets' have been controversial, and this is one aspect of complementary therapies that the NHS has *not* taken to its heart.

There are many forms of 'health' diet, some based on complex philosophies or religions. One alternative is Gerson Therapy, after the ideas of Dr Max Gerson. His diet consists mainly of raw or steamed fruit and fresh vegetables. Macrobiotic diets, based on ancient Chinese philosophies of yin and yang, are also used in treating cancer. This kind of diet aims to restore balance using whole grains, vegetables, fish, beans, nuts and fruits.

But diet is always a minefield and when it comes to cancer there are baffling contradictions between the various kinds. Some are expensive and awkward to follow without a great deal of family support. Others may mean radical changes, weight loss and – doctors fear – weakening of the cancer patient. And unfortunately women already have a tendency to become consumed with guilt over diets because of the enormous pressures we face when it comes to food and our bodies.

The Bristol Centre has acknowledged these issues and, after more than a decade of experience, has revised its diet to make sure that women aren't subject to extra stresses as a result of trying to follow a diet that is difficult and expensive, and which isolates them at family mealtimes. Their new approach is to make gentle changes in diet, enjoying and exploring food, rather than turning eating into a penance.

They have published the following guidelines:

Recommended foods:

- Wholefood (i.e. nothing added or taken away) such as wholemeal bread and brown rice.
- Fresh fruit and vegetables (not tinned or frozen), especially green leafy ones like cabbage, broccoli, sprouts.
- Raw food – salads – vegetables, fruit and raw cereals (muesli), nuts, seeds, etc. Try to eat some each day.
- Organically grown food, as available and if affordable.
- Fish and poultry (and game). Deep-sea fish is preferable, as is organically raised poultry.
- High fibre foods such as beans, pulses, lentils, vegetables and cereals.

- Olive oil for cooking. Otherwise cold-pressed oils.
- Variety. Avoid depending on any one food excessively.
- Alcohol – in moderation and preferably of good quality.

Avoid (as much as possible):

- Red meat such as beef, pork, lamb, veal and bacon.
- Caffeine, as in tea, coffee, chocolate and cola drinks.
- Sugar.
- Salt.
- Fats and dairy produce.
- Smoked or pickled foods.
- Preservatives and additives.
- Mouldy or damaged food.

The Bristol Centre also recommends a range of extra vitamins and minerals that are known to help the body in its role of fighting cancer and preventing further recurrence. The Centre says that vitamins and minerals not only support the immune system and weaken cancer cells, but they can enhance the effects of chemotherapy and radiotherapy as well as reducing their side-effects. They can also help the body to heal well after surgery.

Exploring the alternatives

While the Bristol Centre is an acknowledged pioneer in the cancer field, there are other centres for complementary health care and many individual practitioners. It is impossible to generalize about how much complementary therapies will cost. Many practitioners operate a sliding scale of fees, depending upon income.

Increasingly, complementary therapies are available free within the NHS. The charity CancerLink has a directory of cancer centres and self-help groups and their information officers will deal with enquiries by telephone or by post. (CancerLink also has a telephone helpline for Hindi and Bengali speakers.)

Maxine Rosenfield, CancerLink's information service manager, has noticed an 'enormous advance' of complementary therapies within the NHS in the early 1990s, and many hospitals now offer these therapies. However, these tend to be the therapies perceived as 'safe' by conventional doctors, explains Ms Rosenfield, such as aromatherapy and counselling – as opposed to dietary therapies, homeopathy or massage therapies.

Along with the Hammersmith Hospital, the Mount Vernon Hospital in Hertfordshire has recognized the need for complementary therapies and now has its own Cancer Support Centre. The Royal Shrewsbury Hospital (NHS) also has the Hamar Cancer Help Centre within its grounds. Private cancer help centres, some along the lines of the Bristol Centre, are also available in Edinburgh, Aylesbury, Leighton Buzzard and Letchworth.

Apart from these centres, there are also many self-help groups on the CancerLink directory which include people who are trained in complementary therapies. Many healers, aromatherapists and acupuncturists practise their skills within these groups.

Some of the best-known 'natural' remedies used for breast cancer include homeopathy, the Bach flower remedies, coffee and herb enemas (to flush toxins from the body), as well as iscador and amygdalin.

Iscador is an anthroposophic remedy which is extracted from mistletoe. (Anthroposophy is a twentieth-century alternative approach to medicine which emphasizes the spiritual and emotional aspects of humanity.) Iscador is said to stimulate the immune response and it has been used in breast cancer treatments. GPs can prescribe iscador (by injection or by mouth) on the recommendation of an anthroposophic doctor or homeopath.

Amygdalin (also known as laetrile or B17) is more controversial, and it is illegal in some parts of the US. It is extracted from fruit kernels and pips, and includes a cyanide molecule which is said to act on cancer cells. It is not available on the NHS.

Acupuncture and acupressure

These traditional Chinese medicines are used to regulate energy flow throughout the body. Acupuncturists work on the body's energy pathways (meridians) using fine needles, whereas acupressurists use the pressure of the hands and fingers to revitalize health. Both treatments are recognized by many conventional doctors as useful treatments for pain, and they do have a role in cancer treatment.

Exercise

Exercise is recognized by most health systems, ancient and modern, as playing an important part in health and well-being. Regular exercise releases tension and reduces anxiety. You may prefer Western-style 'aerobic' exercise and sports, or you could try the gentler, Eastern forms of exercise like t'ai chi or yoga.

Mental and spiritual techniques

Many religions and cultures (except for our own) have accepted that mind and spirit have a part to play in healing. Increasingly, organizations like the Bristol Cancer Help Centre are teaching techniques to help cancer patients to relax and gain some sense of control over their lives.

In brief, people with cancer are using age-old methods of deep breathing and concentration to clear their minds of the 'chatter' of daily thought. Once they have reached a state of deep relaxation, the next step is to 'visualize' the eradication of the cancer.

Different people prefer different images: some like to picture their own healthy cells as sharks or missiles attacking cancer cells. Others prefer a more peaceful imagery – such as warm beams of sunlight 'drying up' the cancer cells, or streams of water washing them away. As part of the same process, you can repeat 'affirmations' – statements like 'I choose health' – to affirm your will to get well.

Then of course there is good old-fashioned prayer. Non-religious people might prefer to think of this in terms of positive thinking. Whatever your beliefs it can be very comforting to a patient, and also very helpful to family and friends of a breast cancer sufferer, to feel that they are part of a community of psychological or spiritual support.

The author, Audre Lorde, woke from her mastectomy operation with a sense that the hospital was:

> wrapped in a web of woman love and strong wishes of faith and hope for the whole time I was there, and it made self-healing more possible, knowing I was not alone. Throughout the hospitalization and for some time after, it seemed that no problem was too small or too large to be shared or handled.

Dr Susan Love, the American breast surgeon and author, writes with a warm appreciation of the full range of healing methods available to women with breast cancer. In her book she writes of one of her breast cancer patients who used every resource to heal herself. This patient was a Catholic who, after surgery and a course of tamoxifen, went on a macrobiotic diet, used meditation and visualization, visited Lourdes and attended psychic healing ceremonies. She also carried an amethyst and a rosary made from crystals.

From a state of debilitation caused by secondary cancer in her bone marrow, this woman had taken to mountain-climbing and skiing and dancing. Susan Love comments:

> I don't know which component of this patient's healing work is doing the most good ... But I do know that her commitment to taking control of her healing process has turned a terrifying experience into a triumphant challenge. She is giving herself every chance to survive, and to live a fine, intense life ... Everyone can learn from her example, and use whatever techniques best suit them to make a wholehearted commitment to life.

13
Cosmetic surgery

Cosmetic surgery can be an important aspect of health care for women who have had breast cancer. This chapter looks at the practicalities of cosmetic breast operations, and at how women who have lost a breast feel about further surgery.

Many of the techniques used in breast reconstruction after mastectomy or lumpectomy are fundamentally the same as those used in purely cosmetic operations. (Women's experiences of having their breasts made larger or smaller are explored in Chapter Three.)

The commonest type of cosmetic breast surgery is augmentation, and in the UK about half of these operations are performed on women who have had a breast removed. The other cosmetic techniques, such as breast reduction, can also be carried out to help women look 'normal' after cancer surgery (matching 'normal' breasts with new breasts) – as well as for straightforward cosmetic reasons.

Do women want breast reconstruction?

Some women do want cosmetic surgery after losing a breast to cancer. Others do not. But whatever their point of view, women should surely be given the choice.

As it stands, too many women are still being sent home from British hospitals minus a breast and without counselling or advice on how to deal with this loss. 'Buy a bag of birdseed and put it in your bra' was the only suggestion offered by her doctor to one mastectomy patient. 'Roll up your knickers and stuff them in your bra' is another piece of 'advice' which was given to one woman after surgery.

Yet, according to the authoritative King's Fund Forum, all women should be given the option of reconstructive surgery after mastectomy. In breast units which have the expertise, reconstructions can be done at the same time as the original operation. Other hospitals should offer them at a later date.

Those who have mastectomies without reconstructions should always be given advice about a prosthesis by their surgeon, and an experienced female member of staff should be available to help with its selection and fitting.

Some women feel very strongly that they will feel better, sooner, if the signs of surgery are hidden:

> I don't think I would have coped as well, as quickly, if I hadn't had the implant. It's not identical to what was there before, but it wasn't just a flat surface. For me, because it's been so normal, that's helped me not to even think about it so much.

> The reconstruction was terribly important to me. I did have to ask for it – it wasn't really offered. It's essential to feel you have control over something in your life. When [breast cancer] happens to you,

you feel you aren't in control. With reconstruction, or complementary medicine, or a change in diet, you feel you are doing something apart from what the medical profession is doing. (Breast cancer survivors speaking to the *Guardian*, 20.10.92)

Many doctors believe that women should have reconstructions for the sake of their self-image. In one study, a quarter of women had not let their husbands see them naked after a mastectomy. As Anthony Nash, a surgeon at the Royal Marsden Hospital in London, told the Breast Care Campaign:

None of my patients leaves hospital with one breast. If women tell their friends they have awful scars, their friends won't come forward. Scars [after lumpectomy] should not show. Surgery can be carried out without mutilations. It can be done and it should be done.

According to the surgeon Michael Baum, most patients who want reconstructive surgery are

young and intelligent women who place great importance on their body image and on the significance of their breasts ... [Their] denial, anger and sorrow at the loss of the breast may be alleviated and shortened by the procedure of immediate breast reconstruction.

But even today, when millions of 'healthy' women have had implant surgery to 'improve' their breasts, it is not the norm in this country to offer women reconstructions. Like other breast treatments, this is a matter of pot luck and where you live. (Even surgeons may have to cast about for help on this issue: the Breast Care Campaign has had inquiries from surgeons about where to get a reconstruction for patients.)

Life priority

But in spite of what we might expect – given the enormous sexual emphasis on breasts in our culture – the loss of a breast is not actually the greatest worry that faces a woman with breast cancer. According to Lesley Fallowfield, far more women (60 per cent) are more afraid of cancer itself. Only one in ten women with breast cancer says that losing a breast is her chief concern.

The argument that lumpectomy, which is more conservative surgery, alleviates a woman's mental pain over breast cancer has also been challenged by recent research from the Glasgow Western Infirmary and from the Christie Hospital in Manchester. This study found that, a year after their operations, women's attitudes to their appearance, their enjoyment of sex and their experience of anxiety and depression were about the same – whether they had had a breast removed or not.

A third of the women in this study suffered from depression, and up to a half suffered from anxiety – but only one in ten expressed great concern about her body image. More of an issue than losing a breast was the great need for counselling and support, before and after breast surgery.

Lesley Fallowfield has come to a similar conclusion. Women's greatest fears centre not around mastectomy, but around 'being stigmatized, rejected and dying a lonely, painful and undignified death,' she writes. And these are issues that women face regardless of their surgical treatment.

There are also women who simply don't want breast reconstruction after mastectomy. If this makes people uneasy, perhaps it is because they want breast cancer patients to look 'normal', for reasons to do with the fear of this disease?

Saying 'no' to reconstruction

Many women want neither a device nor an operation to hide the loss of their breast, and some feel resentful about the idea of implants, as well as the expectation that they should wear a prosthesis. 'They feel it's not for them,' says one Breast Cancer Care worker, 'that it's for men.'

Even women who have been told at the time of their mastectomy that they are entitled to come back later for a breast reconstruction tend not to take up the offer. In the year or so they need to wait before reconstruction they often learn to live with their new shape, and can't face the idea of more surgery.

There are also the health risks of breast reconstruction to consider. In recent years much information about the potential hazards of silicone implants has come to light (see Chapter Three). These may harden, rupture or migrate into the armpit. There is a risk of new infections, and a chance that the body may reject the implant. Many women have complained that their 'new' breasts feel hard and unnatural. And there is the possibility that a reconstructed breast may hide signs of a recurrence of cancer.

Furthermore, breast reconstruction means more surgery, not less, at a time when the trend is against any unnecessary surgery. It also implies a justification of mastectomy: if people feel that a breast can be 'reconstructed', perhaps its loss is not such a trauma in the first place?

Other women have taken a stand against breast reconstruction for political and personal reasons. Audre Lorde's book, *The Cancer Journals*, gives a powerful and moving account of her battle to overcome breast cancer. She decided within days of her operation that to disguise the effects of her surgery was a damaging kind of silence, a collusion with a sexist culture which values women for no more than their appearance. Either Lorde would learn to love her own body one-breasted or, she felt, would remain for ever alien to herself.

'Good for morale'? Whose morale?

Yet when Lorde went to visit her surgeon she was told she should wear a prosthesis as to go without was bad for the morale of his office:

> Here we were, in the offices of one of the top surgeons in New York City. Every woman there either had a breast removed, or was afraid of having to have a breast removed. And every woman there could have used a reminder that having one breast did not mean that her life was over, nor that she was less of a woman, nor that she was condemned to the use of a placebo in order to feel good about herself or the way she looked.

Diane Hunter, interviewed by the *Guardian* (20.10.92) after her mastectomy, also experienced pressure to conform:

> The human body is not symmetrical. It's not perfect. It has curves, lumps and angles which make the individual unique. But it's hard to hold onto this view sometimes when the male-dominated medical profession assume that you want 'reconstruction'. 'A young woman like you with young children really ought to go for a silicone implant.' Why? . . . I feel content with my appearance. What causes me pain is when people feel uncomfortable around me because I have not resorted to stuffing my bra with a prosthesis . . . Just let each individual woman cope and come to terms with it in

her own unique way. And let people not flinch when they see an uneven T-shirt.

Just as women are breaking the old taboos by going public about their breast cancer, so some women are rejecting the social pressure to 'hide' their physical loss. Why, they ask, should they mourn in secret? Why should the life and death issues they face be masked in cosmetic concerns? Why should their own struggle to survive be reduced to the level of wearing 'normal' bras or looking good in a swimsuit?

There is an argument too that this process of 'denial' also prevents women confronting the political realities of cancer. When cancer is made invisible, we are less likely to ask questions: What causes it? What can we do to stop it? How should we be treating it? And if the appearance of breasts is perceived to be so important, how are women to overcome their fear of this disease? How will we improve our rates of early detection and treatment?

Yet refusing reconstruction and prostheses is not necessarily 'right' in a society which does put such an emphasis on the 'perfect' breast. Every woman needs to choose her own way of dealing with mastectomy: we have enough guilt on our plates without added guilt over reconstruction or prosthesis. In a world where women are judged by their appearance, it can really help to look 'normal' – whatever the political rights and wrongs of the situation. Some women are also deeply averse to attracting what they perceive as voyeurism in other people by allowing their asymmetry to show.

Many women will make their own decisions on these personal and practical grounds. Perhaps more important than anything else is for a woman to make her own choice on the basis of the best possible information, enabling her to be comfortable with her own body.

Cosmetic surgery: the facts

Breast reconstruction

Breast reconstruction can be done either at the same time as the operation to remove a cancer, or it can be done some time afterwards. The result won't look the same as the original breast, and Breast Cancer Care recommend that women should ask for photographs of a surgeon's previous work before choosing to have reconstruction.

A common form of breast reconstruction uses the silicone implant, which is a thin bag filled with silicone gel. The implant is inserted either beneath the skin of the chest or under the muscle of the chest.

The operation is usually performed under a general anaesthetic and involves a few days in hospital. Apart from pain following the operation, there can be other problems with implants – as detailed in Chapter Three. Silicone implants sometimes harden, and women may have to go through more surgery to replace them.

Another type of reconstruction uses an inflatable silicone bag beneath the chest muscle which, over a period of weeks, is filled with a saline solution. This procedure gradually stretches the skin covering the implant. In one version of this operation the bag stays in place; in another, the bag is replaced by a permanent silicone implant under general anaesthetic.

An alternative technique for reconstructing the breast uses a flap of skin and muscle from the back or abdomen (a myocutaneous flap). The healthy tissue is stitched into the breast, and sometimes a silicone implant is used as well. This is a major operation which leaves scars on the back or abdomen, as well as on the breast. As with all major operations, this one carries a risk of complications.

The nipple and areola can also be reconstructed (usually at a later date) using a skin graft from the thigh or labia for the areola, and a part of the opposite nipple to make a new nipple. It is also possible to buy stick-on nipples, which can be moulded to match the opposite nipple.

Breast Cancer Care has a leaflet called 'Breast Reconstruction' which gives details of these operations.

Breast reduction

This is a more complicated procedure than breast augmentation and leaves more noticeable scars. Areas of the breast are removed symmetrically and the nipple and areola are transplanted upwards. This means that the nerve endings to the nipple as well as the milk ducts are cut, making breastfeeding impossible and often leaving nipples feeling numb.

The operation is performed under general anaesthetic and usually involves a four-day stay in hospital. It takes some four weeks to recover fully from the operation and a supporting bra has to be worn day and night for about six weeks.

Finding a surgeon

As with so many other aspects of breast care, good cosmetic surgeons are in short supply and not always easy to find. So beware: this is a field sometimes exploited by doctors who may be more interested in your money than in your best interests.

If you have already had breast surgery for cancer, your consultant surgeon may know of a good surgeon either in the NHS or in private practice. If you are looking for purely cosmetic surgery, again, your GP may be able to refer you to a good surgeon. Breast reconstruction after cancer should be available on the NHS. Purely cosmetic surgery is sometimes available, at your doctor's discretion. Private clinics may charge several thousand pounds for surgery.

If your doctor doesn't know of anybody, ask him or her to write to the British Association of Plastic Surgeons (BAPS), or alternatively the British Association of Aesthetic Plastic Surgeons (BAAPS).

BAPS has a list of members who are experts in reconstructive surgery. BAAPS has members who specialize in the more cosmetic aspects of plastic surgery. BAAPS will send a list of members and a fact sheet if you write to them with a stamped, addressed A5 envelope. You then take this list to your own GP for advice and a referral letter.

14
Tales of breast cancer

Breast cancer has profound effects, not only on the lives of the women who discover they have it, but on the lives of the people they love and who love them. For every woman with breast cancer, there are many more sisters and daughters, husbands and lovers, friends and relatives who may also be knocked sideways by the diagnosis.

First reactions

Women who have had breast cancer often say that the worst part of the whole experience is the fear they feel in the early days before a definite diagnosis. As one woman told the counsellor and psychologist Lesley Fallowfield:

> It was a living nightmare, that three weeks – knowing what it was but not knowing for sure. Thinking it might be cancer and it spreading everywhere was all I could do night and day. Nothing has happened since – the mastectomy or the radiotherapy treatment sessions – that were as bad as that time.

None the less, to most women the cancer diagnosis still comes as a dreadful shock, and the following days can bring a range of confusing emotions ranging from fear and bewilderment to anger and disbelief.

Some women want to talk about it. Others don't. Many fear mastectomy, fear being 'less of a woman' after breast surgery, and, of course, there is fear of death. The photographer Jo Spence recalled how the news affected her in her book *Putting Myself in the Picture*:

> The [knowledge] that now, I could lose first one, then another breast, terrified me beyond all reason, beyond anything that had ever happened before.

Women with children may also feel devastated by the prospect of not being there as their children grow up:

> The very worst thing was having a fifteen-month-old daughter and thinking, 'This girl won't have a mum'. I just assumed the worst while I waited for the tests on my lymph nodes to come back. There was no counselling, and the overriding feeling was one of loneliness. (*Guardian*, 20.10.92)

Once cancer has been confirmed, everything seems to happen very quickly – perhaps too quickly. The shock is of the level of a major bereavement. Yet within days there may also be a disfiguring operation, followed by medical therapies which can cause sickness and the loss of a woman's hair.

A time of stress

Lizzie was in her mid-thirties and going through a very stressful time when she discovered 'a hard little pea' in her breast:

I went to my GP who sent me for a mammogram. I was told that it was a cyst and it was likely to disperse. My daughter was born soon afterwards, and when I had stopped breastfeeding the lump was still there – but it had changed into a larger mass. My GP sent me to a specialist and I went into hospital to have the 'cyst' removed.

Two weeks after the operation I got a phone call asking me to come in and see the specialist. As I sat there, topless, he said to me, 'It's more than likely that you've got breast cancer.' He gave me no other information apart from offering me a cosmetic operation to 'replace' my breast, which he specializes in for 'women of my age'. He assumed that my main worry was my appearance, but I wanted to know about the cancer. I was in shock – I felt I was floating – and I felt very isolated. When the doctor had gone I was left with the nurse, who hugged me and said, 'Remember there are lots of ways to get rid of cancer these days.'

Lizzie drove herself home, told her husband and called the Bristol Cancer Help Centre, who urged her to ring her doctor and get her diagnosis confirmed. In due course, Lizzie went into hospital for a lumpectomy followed by radiotherapy, while also following a complementary treatment programme through the Bristol Centre:

I used homeopathy, Bach flower remedies and diet to combat the cancer. My GP was brilliant: he got all the vitamins I needed on prescription, said that he had seen many women recover from cancer and told me my cancer was one of the least aggressive types.

Lizzie says that she was not afraid of dying, but that she battled with a different kind of fear:

It was the fear that comes with not knowing, with not being given information, with worrying that they would treat me like a loony for using complementary therapies. They treat you as if you can't cope with being told the facts. The radiotherapy unit – in a big city hospital – horrified me, and rather than staying in the hospital all week I was taken there daily by a rota of friends. I wanted to live at home, to eat good food, see the blossoms on the trees and watch my daughter learning to walk. But although some of the medical staff were excellent, others had no understanding of what I needed. I felt that I was struggling against negative forces – but it worked because I let all our friends and the Bristol Centre help us.

In contrast to Lizzie, 62-year-old Gwen's cancer was discovered by the National Breast Screening Programme:

After going for screening I received a letter asking me to return for further investigations: it came as a shock. I had a feeling that there was something wrong with me, but I had put it down to stress. I had to wait a month for the appointment, which was unnerving. The worst thing was telling my eldest daughter (aged forty), who was very upset. She just couldn't handle it (I felt that it was because her father had died when she was a teenager), and it was six months before she came to see me. Although I have a very strong relationship with my (second) husband, I didn't want to tell him either. His reaction was most irrational; he felt so much anger.

Gwen had a lumpectomy (a third of her breast was removed) followed by radiotherapy, and although she says the individual doctors and nurses were very kind, the hospital system was hopelessly overstretched:

When I went in for my operation they kept us waiting; they lost my notes; they changed me from one ward to another and they told a friend who came to see me that I wasn't there. They even forgot to give us breakfast. The staff were all terribly overworked and it felt like you were on a conveyor belt.

The results of the operation, in which a third of Gwen's breast was removed, looked worse than she had expected:

It was a bit of a shock when I looked at it. There were no bandages, just a substance like Clingfilm. But you can't dwell on these things: I am a fighter and I prefer to release the tension by making light of things. I joked with my husband that I had a melon on one side and an orange on the other. In the hospital you meet people who are far worse off than yourself and there is a lot of support and friendship. The staff used to tell us off on our [radiotherapy] ward for making so much noise laughing.

The emotional roller-coaster

Many women do have feelings of euphoria after their surgery (they have survived!), but euphoria can dissipate fast as shock and denial wear off. In the months that follow, anxiety, insomnia, anger and depression are common.

Up to a third of women still have psychological and sexual problems one to two years later. Up to 40 per cent of women suffer a depressive illness after mastectomy. Single women, who may be more isolated and who may fear that their sexual attractiveness has gone, are especially vulnerable.

Anxiety can be a problem particularly for women who have had 'conservation' rather than a full mastectomy. They may worry that the disease is returning to their breast. The business of going back to the hospital for follow-up visits can also be an ordeal, bringing back old fears and feelings of dread that the cancer may be back. As one mastectomy patient, interviewed in the *Guardian* (20.10.92) put it, 'You have to go back quite a lot for check-ups in the beginning, and every time you get very nervous and think you've got all sorts of pains.'

The prospect of cancer returning at any time is one of the

cruellest aspects of this disease. This woman told the *Guardian* how she coped when she discovered her second malignant lump:

> Three years ago I had another lump in the same breast and another lumpectomy, which I took very calmly. But you never know whether the cancer is completely gone away. It's quite possible that cells have broken away and gone somewhere else in the body, so whenever I have an unexplained little pain or twinge, I think, – 'This is it.' I don't think you ever really get back to the state you were in before.

Family feelings

Breast cancer affects not only the women who develop it in their bodies, but their sisters and mothers, their husbands and partners, their parents and children, too.

Audre Lorde describes in her book how her daughter reacted to the news of her mother's breast cancer:

> My daughter Beth cried in the waiting room after I told her I was going to have a mastectomy. She said she was sentimentally attached to my breasts. Adrienne (a friend) comforted her, somehow making Beth understand that hard as this was, it was different for me than if I had been her age, and that our experiences are different.

Women who have had mastectomies say that it is very important to let children see what has happened to their mother's body – otherwise their fears and fantasies may run riot. Says one such woman:

> My four-year-old daughter had always bathed with me. After the mastectomy, she came into the bathroom, looked at me, and

wouldn't get into the bath with me. Eventually she said, 'I did prefer you with two.' It took about four months, but she did get into the bath with me again.

Women who have lost their mothers to breast cancer during childhood may suffer deep psychological damage, as well as a lasting fear about their own risks of developing the disease. According to an American book, *Challenging the Breast Cancer Legacy*, which is written for women with breast cancer in their families, these women may have lasting feelings of being abandoned and motherless. As women reach the age at which their mothers became ill, the anxieties can intensify. There may be a fear of ending up like their mothers.

In women who are already adults when their mothers become ill, the trauma tends to be less intense because by adulthood most girls have established a sense of independent self and identity. But if there are conflicts between mothers and daughters, illness is likely to sharpen them. We like to think that crisis will make us noble and that we can transcend our petty differences when disaster strikes. This may be true at first, but once the initial shock has passed, old family patterns tend to repeat themselves within the new framework of illness.

On the other hand loving relationships between mothers and daughters can become even more loving. As one mother told her daughters, 'It could have been worse: it could have been one of you.'

Bad feelings

Breast cancer is a disease which can bring tremendous feelings of guilt, blame and shame in people connected to the woman who is ill, as well as in the woman who has been diagnosed.

According to one nurse counsellor who has worked in this field for many years, husbands will often privately ask her if they are to blame for their wives' cancers. They worry in retrospect that rough sex play – or even sexual violence – may have caused the tumour. (Cancer cannot be caused this way, although other physical trauma can result.)

Family members may also be stricken with guilty feelings for a variety of reasons. The simple fact of the blood tie – and knowledge that breast cancer appears to run in families – may be enough:

> My father thought it was all his fault because his sister and his mother had both had breast cancer. In a strange way, I actually felt better about that – first because both had survived, and had lived a long time after having the disease; and also because it meant that it wasn't my fault, there was nothing I could have done to prevent it. (Helena McCloskey, *Guardian*, 20.10.92)

For sisters of women with breast cancer there can be a welter of disturbing feelings to deal with, especially if a mother has had cancer too. Sisters often feel great guilt. A sister is someone who is closer to you physically – and probably emotionally, too – than anyone else on earth. When she discovers she has breast cancer you may feel, 'Why her and not me?' Or even more painfully, because we all have a powerful wish to live, 'I'm glad it wasn't me.'

Sisters – as well as daughters – of women with breast cancer may respond with immediate concern and tenderness in the early days of their relatives' illness. They may suppress their own fears – or feel guilty and selfish when these fears surface. But sooner or later sisters and daughters will probably have to face the knowledge that they are at higher risk of the disease themselves, with all the anxiety, regret and anger that may bring. They are powerful feelings that can affect a woman's attitude to her own body and her own womanhood for the rest of her life.

Support and affection

What can help women survive this time emotionally? The affection and loyalty of partners, friends and family is a tremendous help in pulling women through. A good relationship with doctors and nurses also makes a positive difference (unfortunately there is, as yet, no routine service which offers counselling in all hospitals) and a good support group or network can be invaluable:

> During those bleak days, only other women cancer patients made any sense to me. Suddenly my phone was ringing off the hook with calls from complete strangers, consoling me as I sobbed my heart out. Cancer networking was the only thing that got me through those first six months. (Kathy Evans in the *Guardian*, 20.10.92)

Breast cancer can put relationships under enormous strain, and reactions from male partners of women who have mastectomies can vary from the lovingly supportive to the downright callous. This Breast Cancer Care worker has seen some very sad situations:

> I've met women whose husbands have left them after mastectomy. It may be the last straw in a failing marriage, but she feels *that's why*. It adds to the wife's distress.

Another woman had worked all her life as a midwife, yet difficulties in her faltering marriage stopped her from getting the medical attention she knew that she needed:

> I found my breast lump before my ex-husband moved out and I didn't do anything about it. I couldn't face up to the possibility of mastectomy with him there. He was what you would call a 'breast man'. He couldn't have coped if I'd lost a breast. As soon as he was gone I was able to deal with it.

On the other hand, relationships that are already strong can be strengthened even further by the experience of cancer. Some men, as many women who have had breast cancer testify, become especially sensitive and supportive when the women they love are at risk. And many women say that their surgery makes little or no difference to their sexual relationships. Says Lizzie:

> It didn't worry me. I like clothes and so on, but my husband's interest is in *me* and not in my 'glamour'.

Lizzie is now forty-seven and after ten years of check-ups she is officially 'in the clear':

> The whole experience of breast cancer has changed me. It has sorted me out and made me find myself. I am just Lizzie now: what matters is who I am and not what I do. And I really value my family: the most important thing is *us*.

Gwen is still recovering from the side-effects of radiotherapy (she is still very sore, with aching arm muscles) and she is on tamoxifen. Her prognosis is good: as with many cancers discovered by screening, hers was very small. And she, too, says the experience has changed her:

> I am more 'selfish' now. I don't put off too much and I don't let my husband have his way so much! I have gone back to work and I keep in touch with the friends I made in hospital. I would have liked counselling, but there was none in our town, so instead we meet and talk amongst ourselves. I am looking forward and very much making the most of everything.

15
The politics of breast care

In the end, the way that our breast health problems are treated cannot be separated from the way we think of breasts – and the way we think of women.

The people with the power to make the decisions about breast care – whether as doctors, health administrators or politicians – are mostly men. But the people with most at stake in breast care are women. Would breast health be in its current confused and neglected state if it were a male problem? Would we continue to have the world's worst record of deaths from breast cancer if the sufferers were men?

Increasingly, women are emerging from private grief to express public anger at the breast cancer death toll. As the paediatrician Dr Daphne Pearson told *Vogue* (January 1993), breast cancer has long suffered from being a 'woman's disease' – and a disease of older women too:

> It hasn't been taken seriously. There has been this feeling that it gets a few women who die after their children are grown up. It doesn't matter that much.

Paradoxically, the ageist bias could now begin to work in women's favour as people begin to think of breast cancer as a younger women's disease too. Once, it was an unmentionable illness that one's grandmother had tried to keep a secret until she died. These days many more younger women are quite open about having the disease, and women in the public eye – from Betty Ford to Gloria Steinem to 'Green Goddess' Diana Moran – have raised its profile. Earlier detection and screening are also lowering the age at which women are diagnosed.

But for too long, when it comes to breasts, prejudices have been working against women's interests. Women with breast pain are still accused of being 'neurotic' by their doctors. Women who ask questions about their treatments are still labelled 'hysterical'. Too often we meet with the attitude that 'doctor knows best' and women's deep feelings about how we are treated are ignored.

These attitudes cause problems in all aspects of breast care, but the most urgent problems are in breast cancer care.

Better care in Bombay?

Authorities on breast cancer are using the word 'epidemic'. The disease is now the biggest killer of women in their middle years in Britain. Across Europe it represents the single biggest risk to women's health.

Yet in Britain the national picture for breast care remains lamentable – with occasional glimpses of excellence. And because no one has properly recorded that picture, or compared treatments across the country, women find it virtually impossible to get the best care for themselves.

Ideally, every woman with a breast disease should have access to a specialist team. Yet no comparable country has fewer specialists. The most common breast problems are benign. However in 1993, Breast Care Campaign counted only five specialist breast pain clinics in the country – in Nottingham, Cardiff, Dundee, Edinburgh and at Guy's Hospital in London.

As for breast cancer, a *Sunday Express* investigation in January 1993 revealed that, proportionately, Britain has sixteen times fewer cancer physicians than the US. Even Costa Rica has three times more specialists per head of population.

Professor Karol Sikora, director of clinical oncology at the Hammersmith Hospital in London, told the *Sunday Express*:

> For all the relative wealth of this country, it is quite possible that cancer patients may have a worse chance of survival in Bodmin than in Bombay. Three thousand women die unnecessarily each year because too many patients have no chance to see a specialist and subsequently may not be prescribed the correct drugs or treatment for their particular case.

In Britain, we have the worst recorded survival rate for breast cancer in the world. Only 58 per cent of British women with breast cancer live beyond five years – compared to 73 per cent in the US, 72 per cent in France, 68 per cent in Norway and 66.5 per cent in East Germany.

NHS overwhelmed

There may be other reasons for these figures – many British women don't come for medical treatment until their cancers are dangerously advanced – but the shortage of specialists is a major factor. The NHS funds less than twenty posts for consultant cancer physicians in Britain. Fifty-three further posts are funded by cancer research organizations.

British consultants may see five times as many new cancer patients a year as their colleagues in other European countries. Lack of expert care means that women with breast cancer aren't getting the time and meticulous treatment they need. Doctors are saying that the health service is overwhelmed, that services are fragmented and no one takes responsibility for coordinating women's care.

In the breast cancer literature (the kind that is put together by women), horror stories abound of women being told 'not to worry' by one doctor, and 'it's malignant' by another. Again, many women are told they 'must' have a mastectomy, but when they object or question their doctors, they end up with lumpectomies or other treatments.

Many women are operated on by general surgeons without much experience in breast surgery. These surgeons often see mastectomy as the easiest, safest and cheapest way of dealing with breast cancer. The latest techniques in breast conservation are beyond their expertise. Women may not be referred for radiotherapy: if they are, the radiotherapist may not know whether chemotherapy is required.

Women who live in London, where many cancer specialists are concentrated, have a far better chance of seeing a specialist than women who live elsewhere. Breast cancer patients in the north-west are said to have only a one-in-three chance of seeing a specialist before they die. Since the restructuring of the NHS, many women have lost the option of travelling to a specialist centre for treatment – even if they have been able to work out how to find one.

From the medical point of view, scientists and doctors are calling for change. Professor Barry Gusterson from the Institute of Cancer Research wants to see 'a group of internationally respected experts who will produce guidelines' for the best treatments. He believes we should also be carrying out national surveys about current treatments to assess what changes are necessary.

From a woman's point of view we must have this kind of basic information if we are to be able to make informed choices in breast care treatment. The time is right for a *Good Breast Care Guide*, assessing treatments and women's experience of these across the country.

It is up to women to insist on these changes. And Barry Gusterson doubts that men will see breast health as a priority unless women take the initiative:

> Governments don't do anything (in this field) unless they are forced to do it. To make them shift we need campaigns like those organized by women in America.

How much do we care?

Breast cancer surgeons and scientists are increasingly sticking their heads above the parapet and making noises about the lack of coordination and the lack of government funding for breast cancer. Barry Gusterson puts it like this:

> The amount spent annually on initiatives to find the cause of breast cancer is less than that which is put into the launch of a new brand of soap powder. Are these really our priorities?
>
> In this country, the government is letting charities pick up the bill. Breast cancer funding is done on a pot-luck basis. There is no strategy. We need a proper look at it – as we would in industry. We should identify the need, cost it and do it.

Ian Fentiman, deputy director of the ICRF-funded cancer research unit at Guy's Hospital in London, has also expressed his frustration at the lack of input into breast cancer. He told *Elle* magazine:

> The government doesn't do anything. Cancer research in this country is virtually privatized with most of it being done by the CRC and the ICRF. The government gives a certain amount to the Medical Research Council – but it's just not enough.
>
> The screening service is done on a shoestring and I'm worried that it could be made locally funded and we could end up with regional authorities saying they can't afford the luxury of it. We need much more money for research – the charities have been hit by the recession like everyone else – and there is a lot of clinical research we want to do but can't because we have had to cut back.

In 1992 the charity 'Breakthrough' was set up to raise £15 million for a specialist research centre in association with the Royal Marsden Hospital and the Institute of Cancer Research. The centre will be a kind of 'research hotel', explains Barry Gusterson, where the best scientists and doctors will focus on breast cancer research, pooling their expertise and working together. Already, British scientists and doctors have been raising their horizons and making links with colleagues in Europe and America.

Benign breast disease: also underfunded

Benign breast disease is also starved of research funding in this country. This is an area where drug companies cannot make great profits. Much breast care is preventive, involving change of diet and so on, rather than the use of drugs. And in this country medical research is all too often drug-company led.

This is because governments have been steadily withdrawing funding for research. The Medical Research Council has suffered serious cuts. Inevitably, drug companies have been asked to step in, but their research is goal-directed and linked to potential profits. Professor Robert Mansel, now a world authority on benign breast disease and a staunch supporter of women's right to better care, began his ground-breaking research into breast pain in the early 1970s. He points out that it was university-based:

> If I was starting out now, I wouldn't be able to do the same research. It is very difficult in this country to get funds for benign breast problems.

Barry Gusterson agrees with Mansel's plea for a return to basics:

> We don't even know how the normal breast develops, and this will be a major part of the Breakthrough Centre's programme.

Mansel believes that the future of breast research lies here, and that a greater understanding of benign breast problems could lead to a breakthrough in our understanding of breast cancer. If we knew why breasts get lumpy, if we knew why cells cluster together in the way that they do – then we might be closer to understanding why they get out of control in malignant growths too.

International pressure

Over the years Professor Mansel has been struck by the more sympathetic attitudes to breasts and to breast health in other countries. And international changes to breast health – and, in particular, breast cancer – are now having their impact here.

In America, women have already succeeded in putting breast health high on the political agenda. US pressure groups have made breast cancer a high-profile feminist issue. Gloria Steinem has said that all the gains made in breast health in the past two decades in America have been the result of women's campaigns to end the cruelty of unnecessary surgery (radical mastectomies were routinely performed in spite of evidence that they did nothing to improve a woman's chance of survival).

A campaign at the beginning of the 1990s in the US made great strides in raising public awareness of the disease. Women's groups were galvanized into lobbying Congress to pump millions of dollars into research and cure for the disease. Cori Vancheri of the National Cancer Institute in Washington told the *European* (29.10.92) that as a result of this:

> There is virtually one mammograph machine on every corner. Many of the women who responded to our campaign thought breast cancer was a normal thing. We showed them that they do have choices and that there was something they could do about it.

In 1992 the pressure bore further fruit when the US government switched $200 million in funding from the defence budget directly into breast cancer research.

Initiatives have also been coming from Europe, where the European School of Oncology in Milan (an independent, non-profit body) has launched the international 'Europa Donna' campaign to improve breast care in Europe. One aim was to encourage women to lobby their governments and doctors for better care, with the backing of thousands of other women across Europe.

The European School of Oncology has also urged women to demand that they be treated with modern low-dose mammography equipment by well-trained and experienced staff. Regular screening under these conditions, they argue, can reduce the chances (for women over fifty) of dying of breast cancer by 30 per cent. To date, only women who live in Britain, the Netherlands or Sweden are offered regular screening after the age of fifty.

The European School of Oncology is also encouraging a more sensitive approach to breast surgery and to women in general. Professor Umberto Veronesi, who heads the Europa Donna Campaign, pioneered the lumpectomy operation at the beginning of the 1980s. He argues that techniques are now so sophisticated that few women should have to leave an operating theatre without a breast. Even if the breast had to be removed, as it is in 40 per cent of operations across Europe, it could be reconstructed during the same operation.

This will be greeted by some women as good news. But not all women want the extra surgery of reconstruction after mastectomy. And there are dissenting voices who want more than brilliant surgeons to limit the consequences of breast cancer after it has developed.

They point out that we haven't yet properly addressed the question of *why* so many Western women get breast cancer. We don't even understand the basics of this disease. Any progress made in the past two decades has been a matter of fine-tuning of treatments.

What women want and what women are asking of the medical

profession is a new look at the whole picture of breast disease, together with a change in attitudes towards the breast itself.

Conspiracy of silence?

Death rates from breast cancer have not gone down for more than thirty years. Yet instead of asking, 'Why not?', women are urged to look to their own lifestyles. Have they put their careers before having babies ('selfish')? Have they overindulged in fatty foods ('greedy')? Have they neglected to examine their breasts regularly ('lazy')?

Or have they repressed their emotions? Consumed too much alcohol? Turned too early to the contraceptive pill? Were they guilty of vanity in bottle-feeding to 'keep their figures'?

Women are often quick to take the blame for breast cancer, whereas in reality there is no proof that anything we do makes much difference to our survival. Of course it may help to go to screening appointments, and to examine ourselves: it is possible to detect breast cancer earlier this way and to avoid extra surgery. But there is little we can do to avoid breast cancer. According to the US Centres for Disease Control, three-quarters of all breast cancers occur in women with no obvious risk factors.

Deborah Hutton, writing in *Vogue* (January 1993), believes that there is a conspiracy of silence around this fact, born of medical embarrassment together with a desire to protect women from the bad news. But the time for mutual hand-holding and sympathy amongst women is over, she argues:

The activists' charge that only the truth will jolt us out of our collective inertia, enable all women to profit from the progress that has already been made and expose the way that the less than truthful emphasis on early detection and a healthier lifestyle dumps the burden of the breast cancer on the woman herself, leaving her to find her own answers rather than impelling the whole of society to take the problem on and give it the research priority it deserves.

While women are being blamed for becoming ill, it remains true that the basic research on breast cancer has not been done. Funding – sparse as it is – has concentrated on the profitable end of the business, which is treatment. Governments, argues Deborah Hutton, have been able to avoid some awkward questions:

[questions] about exposure to electromagnetic fields or to environmental pollution, or speculation about whether the same malign influences that have halved men's sperm count and doubled the number of tumours in their testicles and prostate glands over the last half century are also giving rise to malignancies in the female breast.

Hutton cites a study from the University of Connecticut School of Medicine which found higher concentrations of the toxins PCB and DDT in the breast tissue of women who had malignant tumours than in those who had benign breast diseases. These substances are thought to come into the food chain from polluting industries, but rather than tackling this pollution, women are urged to stop eating the fats that harbour pollutants.

Which way now?

We don't yet understand breast disease. We can't yet stop breast cancer. But in changing cultural attitudes, we could revolutionize breast health.

In all that women say about the experience of breast diseases, in all that has been written, one thing stands out. When women complain, they rarely complain of pain. They rarely even complain of disfigurement. What they do complain about is how they are treated as people. The stories which last long after the physical scars have healed are stories of the lack of sensitivity, lack of understanding and lack of empathy – mostly on the part of the medical profession.

According to Andrea Whalley:

> Women do want to be listened to. We do want to be taken seriously and not have our health problems belittled as 'women's problems'. We don't want to be patted on the head and told to 'put up with it', or meet with doctors' assumptions that a lump is a blocked duct and that we are 'neurotic'.
>
> Even if we have made a mistake and all is well, we are never 'wasting a doctor's time'. All of us contribute to that doctor's salary, and the doctor should be as pleased as we are when we do not have a serious problem.

Any serious illness, especially cancer, can bring loneliness and grief in its wake and many women with breast cancer are desperately in need of support and understanding. Says Andrea Whalley:

> There are so many stories of women in their hospital beds, crying, and nobody there to listen to their sorrows and fears. We need

more breast care nurses to make sure that kind of thing doesn't happen.

Women across the breast care field agree that good counselling and emotional support from more specialist nurses would be a tremendous boon. Many callers to the Breast Care Campaign's telephone helpline benefited from being referred to breast care nurses in their area. Although the number of breast care nurses has increased dramatically in the last decade (to 170 in 1993), there are still not nearly enough of these important nurses to go around.

To some extent the range of self-help groups and telephone helplines have been filling the gaps by offering women information and support. Currently there are a number of helplines which deal with inquiries about breast cancer, but none which deals specifically with benign breast problems – although staff at the Breast Care Campaign do their best to help. Funding is also a perennial problem for these groups.

Climate change

But we can't expect the medical profession to shoulder all the responsibilities. There are deeper social and political reasons why other countries care more about the breast, invest more in breast health and breastfeed their babies more comfortably than we do. What can the rest of us do to change the climate which determines breast care?

The media could help, by paying as much attention to benign breast diseases as it does to breast cancer. As important as it is for women to know about breast cancer, it is also important for us to recognize that not every lump is a death sentence.

Better health education, from the earliest school years onwards, would make an enormous difference. If our children could grow up with some understanding about breasts, knowing that they exist for feeding babies as much as for physical pleasure, then we might have less sniggering and shame over breasts as we grow up. And the next generation might avoid the embarrassment that stops British women from going to the doctor with cancer symptoms.

But if we are going to learn about our breasts, becoming 'breast aware', we need the kinds of services that can deal with the problems we discover. Yet there are still areas of this country where women can't get a mammogram, and many more where the technique of fine needle aspiration – vital in diagnosing so many breast diseases – is not available. We need better diagnostic services, as well as better psychological support.

A major step forward would be to open up the services and facilities of the National Breast Screening Programme, so that these would be available to *all* women, not just women over fifty who have been called for screening.

Doctors also need better support (no one counsels surgeons about *their* feelings as they try to care for desperately ill women), as well as clear information. Information about breast cancer will remain confusing until we know more about the disease. But good information about benign breast diseases should not be so hard to come by. According to Professor Mansel:

> The textbooks are not clear about breast problems, and so GPs are not clear about it either.

As a result, doctors go their own way in breast care. (In 1993, Professor Mansel published a paper giving guidelines for GPs in breast care.)

Permission to be human

Women can take a lead in changing the cultural climate, starting with ourselves. We can talk about breasts, challenge the taboos, express our dislike of breast images that upset us and encourage breastfeeding.

We can also stop caring for everyone else at the expense of caring for ourselves. Just as we are too quick to take the blame for our illnesses, we are too ready to protect everyone else from our own feelings. Andrea Whalley thinks women should escape the tyranny of always being the one who copes:

> Women say, 'Don't you worry about me' to our partners, to our children – even to our doctors. We say, 'I'm all right, I'm not upset', when we *are* upset. Women need someone who can say to them – it's all right to be upset. This could be a breast care nurse, it could be a volunteer counsellor. But we must allow ourselves to be human beings and to turn to somebody.

Within the family, denial of our feelings means a lost opportunity for children to learn that loss is a part of life – and that, afterwards, life goes on. Why should we keep our grief to ourselves? It does children no harm to know that their mother feels sadness, because they also see that in time she feels better. In their turn, children will feel able to say when *they* feel sadness and pain. And they are given the opportunity to share with the family in comforting the mother and helping her to recover.

Talking about breasts . . .

Sharing our pain with men could also have a profound impact
on the relationship between the sexes which is at the root of so
many breast care issues. Instead of setting up an expectation
that women are superhuman, or simply pretending that nothing
has happened (some women don't even tell their husbands they
have had a mastectomy), we can ask men for emotional support.
Says Andrea Whalley:

> Some men who treat women badly have never seen their own
> mother in distress because she has shielded them from her pain.
> Women will not do the human race any harm to share their pain:
> it gives their partners permission to be human.

Ultimately, breast health care can't be separated from the
other issues raised in this book. We won't have sensitive and
satisfactory health care until women are allowed to be comfortable with their breasts and until men recognize that breasts are
not just for sex, not just for them. We need to address the whole
picture; unravelling men's mixed feelings of desire, fear and
hatred for breasts; restoring respect for breastfeeding; restoring
respect for women.

Helping Organizations

Breast health

BACUP

3 Bath Place, Rivington Street, London EC2A 3JR

Information Service: Freephone 0800 181199 Mon–Thurs 10am
  to 7pm; Fri 10am to 5.30 pm. London callers: 071 608 1661
Counselling Service (London based): 071 696 9000
Administration: 071 696 9003

BACUP offers medical and non-medical information and support
to cancer patients, their families and friends. The London-based
one-to-one counselling service offers weekly appointments for up
to eight sessions. Services are free and confidential. Publications
include: *Understanding Cancer of the Breast*; *Understanding Secondary Breast Cancer*; *Understanding Radiotherapy* and a *Tamoxifen
factsheet*.

Breakthrough

PO Box 2JP, London W1A 2JP. Tel: 071 405 5111

Breakthrough Breast Cancer is a charity formed to raise £15
million to bring together doctors and scientists from different
disciplines into one centre of excellence which aims to eradicate
breast cancer.

The Breast Care Campaign
1 St Mary Abbots Place, London W8 6LS. Tel: 071 371 1510

Established in 1991, the Breast Care Campaign aims to help all women understand general breast care. It focuses particularly on benign breast disease, providing information and raising awareness among health professionals, women's organizations and the media. Its steering committee has representatives from five major women's health care groups: the Medical Advisory Service, the Premenstrual Society, Women's Health Concern, Women's Nationwide Cancer Control Campaign and the National Council of Women.

Breast Cancer Care
15/19 Britten Street, London SW3 3TZ
Help and Information Line: 071 867 1103
Administration: 071 867 8275

Breast Cancer Care is a national organization offering free help, information and support to women with breast cancer or other breast-related problems. Services include a Helpline, Prosthesis Advisory Service and Volunteer Service. Trained volunteers with personal experience offer one-to-one emotional support.
Breast Cancer Care is also at:

- Suite 2/8, 65 Bath Street, Glasgow G2 2BX.
  Tel: 041 353 1050
- 511 Lanark Road, Edinburgh EH14 5DQ.
  Tel: 031 458 5598 (9–12.30, or answering machine)

Bristol Cancer Help Centre
Grove House, Cornwallis Grove, Clifton, Bristol, Avon BS8 4PG
Tel: 0272 743216

The Bristol Centre offers weekly residential and non-residential holistic courses for cancer patients including counselling, relaxation, visualization, meditation, art therapy, healing, dietary advice and vitamin supplements. Seminars and workshops are also available for specialist groups.

CancerLink
17 Britannia Street, London WC1X 9JN
also at 9 Castle Terrace, Edinburgh, EH1 2DP. Tel: 031 228
   5557
Information Service: 071 833 2451 or 031 228 5557
Asian language line: 071 713 7867

Founded in 1982 by people with personal and professional experience of cancer, this organization provides information and support for people with cancer. The trained staff of CancerLink's Information Service will answer questions about options in health care, enabling people to make informed decisions. Telephone information is provided in English, Hindi and Bengali. CancerLink's Self-Help and Support Service acts as a resource to support and self-help groups and individuals throughout Britain.

CancerLink's 'Directory of Cancer Support and Self-Help' includes details of over 400 support groups across the country. Their register of contacts includes a lesbian network and one for black people. They also produce a range of useful publications on emotional and practical issues about cancer.

RAGE (Radiotherapy Action Group)
c/o Linda Brendon, 30 Bloomhall Road, Upper Norwood, London SE19 1JQ

An action group for people suffering a range of side-effects after radiotherapy.

Complementary health

The British Holistic Medical Association
179 Gloucester Place, London NW1 6DX. Tel: 071 262 5299

The Institute of Complementary Medicine
21 Portland Place, London W1N 3AF. Tel: 071 636 9543

Breastfeeding

Association of Breastfeeding Mothers (ABM)
26 Holmshaw Close, Sydenham, London SE26 4TH.
Tel: 081 778 4769

The ABM is a voluntary organization offering support and encouragement to mothers who choose to breastfeed. ABM counsellors run support groups and they are trained to find solutions to non-medical problems of breastfeeding. All counsellors are mothers who have enjoyed breastfeeding their own babies.

La Lèche League
La Lèche League (GB), BM3424, London WC1N 3XX.
Tel: 071 242 1278

La Lèche League is a charitable organization which aims to provide information, support and encouragement – primarily through personal help – to every woman who wishes to breast-feed her baby. It offers support groups, LLL breastfeeding 'leaders' and a wide range of leaflets and publications.

National Childbirth Trust
Alexandra House, Oldham Terrace, Acton, London W3 6NH.
Tel: 081 992 8637

The NCT is a charity offering information and support in pregnancy, childbirth and early parenthood. It aims to enable parents to make informed choices about such issues as breastfeeding. The NCT has over 500 trained breastfeeding counsellors, plus a range of leaflets on breastfeeding.

Royal College of Midwives
15 Mansfield Street, London W1M OBE.

The RCM's Infant-Feeding Specialist Group may be able to help with inquiries about breastfeeding problems.

Baby Milk Action
BMA, 23 St Andrew's Street, Cambridge CB2 3AX.
Tel: 0223 464420

BMA is an independent, non-profit organization which raises awareness of the dangers of artificial infant feeding and campaigns to protect infant health. It has a small head office in Cambridge plus a network of local groups and area contacts across the UK. It is part of the International Baby Food Action Network (IBFAN).

Breast Surgery

British Association of Aesthetic Plastic Surgeons
The Royal College of Surgeons in England, 35–43 Lincoln's Inn
Fields, London WC2

British Association of Plastic Surgeons
As for the BAAPS.

Glossary

Abscess A painful, boil-like infection under the skin.

Anthroposophy A complementary therapy based on the ideas of Rudolph Steiner.

Areola The circular area of dark skin surrounding the nipple.

Aspiration The withdrawal of fluid from the body using a needle and syringe.

Benign breast disease A range of common, non-cancerous disorders with symptoms such as lumpiness, tenderness and pain.

Benign growth A non-cancerous growth which does not invade other body tissues or spread through the body.

Biopsy The removal of a sample of body tissue which can be closely examined in a laboratory.

Cyst A fluid-filled sac which usually (but not always) feels soft to the touch.

Cytology The study of cells.

Duct A channel in the body for carrying fluid (as in the breast's milk ducts).

Duct ectasia Enlarging and hardening of a diseased duct, together with nipple discharge.

Fat necrosis The death of fat cells, causing a lump in the breast.

Fibroadenoma A non-cancerous growth of fibrous and glandular tissue in the breast.

Fibroadenosis A spread of the condition which causes fibroadenomas.

Fibrocystic disease A term used (in different ways by different doctors) to describe a wide range of non-cancerous breast conditions.

Fine needle aspiration cytology A kind of biopsy in which a small sample of a lump can be taken through a needle (usually without anaesthetic) and then examined for signs of cancer.

Galactocele A type of cyst.

HRT Hormone Replacement Therapy is a hormone treatment given to replace levels of oestrogen in women during or after their menopause.

Lumpectomy The surgical removal of a breast lump.

Lymphoedema Swelling caused by the accumulation of lymph (a body fluid similar to blood) which may follow the removal of the lymph glands under a woman's arms in breast cancer surgery.

Malignant growth A cancerous growth.

Mammogram X-ray of the breast.

Mastalgia Breast pain.

Mastectomy Surgical removal of the breast.

Mastitis Inflammation of the breast, most often found in breast-feeding women.

Montgomery's tubercles Special sweat glands on the areola which secrete the lubricant 'sebum' to protect and soften the nipple during breastfeeding.

Oxytocin A hormone which causes the muscle cells around the milk glands to contract in the 'let-down' reflex, and which is also involved in sexual response.

Paget's disease A rare form of cancer which causes an eczema-like rash on the nipple.

Prolactin Hormone which controls the production of milk in breastfeeding.

Prosthesis A substitute for a part of the body – for instance, a breast form used to fill out a bra after mastectomy.

Secondaries Cancers which have spread into the rest of the body from travelling cells of the primary tumour.

Tamoxifen A hormone therapy for breast cancer, usually in tablet form, which can control the spread of the disease.

Thelarche Growth of breasts at puberty.

Ultrasound A way of scanning body tissues and organs using sound waves.

Bibliography

Balaskas, J. and Gordon, Y., *The Encyclopedia of Pregnancy and Birth*, Macdonald, 1987.

Baum, M., *Breast Cancer*, W. B. Saunders, 1982.

Boston, S. and Louw, J., *Disorderly Breasts*, Camden Press, 1987.

Brohn, P., *Gentle Giants*, Century, 1986.

Brohn, P., *The Bristol Programme*, Century, 1987.

Cirket, C., *A Woman's Guide to Breast Health*, Thorsons, 1992.

Cochrane, J. and Szarewski, A., *Breast Book: A Complete Guide to Breast Health*, Optima, 1989.

Fallowfield, L. and Clark, A., *Breast Cancer*, Routledge, 1991.

Faludi, S., *Backlash: The Undeclared War Against Women*, Chatto & Windus, 1992.

Hite, S., *The Hite Report on Female Sexuality*, 1976.

Hite, S., *The Hite Report on Men and Male Sexuality*, 1981.

Hughes, L.E., Mansel, R.E. and Webster, D., *Benign Disorders and Diseases of the Breast*, Baillière Tindall, 1989.

Kidman, B., *A Gentle Way with Cancer*, Century Arrow, 1986.

Kitzinger, S., *Breastfeeding your Baby*, Dorling Kindersley, 1989.

Lorde, A., *The Cancer Journals*, Sheba Feminist Publishers, 1985.

Love, S., *Dr Susan Love's Breast Book*, New York, Addison Wesley, 1990.

Masters, W.H. and Johnson, V.E., *Human Sexuality*, Scott Foresman, 1988.

Metcalf, A. and Humphries, M., *The Sexuality of Men*, Pluto Press, 1985.

Morris, D., *The Naked Ape*, Jonathan Cape, 1967.

Odent, M., *The Nature of Birth and Breastfeeding*, Bergin & Garvie, 1992.

Palmer, G., *The Politics of Breastfeeding*, Pandora Press, 1993.

Partridge, E., *Dictionary of Slang and Unconventional English*, Routledge, 1991.

Phillips, A. and Rakusen, J. (eds.), *Our Bodies, Ourselves*, Penguin, 1978.

Renfrew, M., Fisher, C. and Arms, S., *Bestfeeding: Getting Breastfeeding Right for You*, Celestial Arts, USA, 1990.

Roth, P., *The Breast*, Jonathan Cape, 1973.

Royal College of Midwives, *Successful Breastfeeding* (Written for health professionals, this book gives up-to-date research behind good practice.)

Schaler, R.R. and Benderly, B.L., *Challenging the Breast Cancer Legacy*, Harper Collins.

Short, C., *Page Three*, Hutchinson Radius, 1991.

Smale, M., *Book of Breastfeeding*, National Childbirth Trust, 1992.

Spence, J., *Putting Myself in the Picture: A Political, Personal and Photographic Autobiography*, Camden Press, 1986.

Stanway, A. and P., *The Breast*, Mayflower, 1982.

Warner, M., *Monuments and Maidens*, Picador, 1987.

Wolf, N., *The Beauty Myth*, Vintage, 1991.

Index

Page numbers in *italic* refer to the illustrations

Write a postscript to this book

Help us find a cure for Breast Cancer

BREAKTHROUGH Breast Cancer has been set
up specifically to create a Breast Cancer Research Centre.
To achieve this, we need £15 million.
With your help, we'll make it.

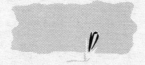

BREAKTHROUGH
BREAST CANCER

PO Box 2JP London W1A 2JP Telephone 071 405 5111 Registered Charity No. 328323 ✂

Name *(block capitals please)* Mrs / Ms / Mr

Address

Postcode

Telephone number (day)   (evening)

I would like to donate

£50 ☐   £25 ☐   £10 ☐   £ _____ ☐ *(tick as appropriate)*

☐ Please send me more information about **BREAKTHROUGH**

☐ I enclose my cheque or postal order made payable to
BREAKTHROUGH Breast Cancer

Please send your completed donation form to:
BREAKTHROUGH Breast Cancer PO Box 2JP, London W1A 2JP Telephone 071 405 5111